Scope AND
Standards
OF PRACTICE

Nursing

2ND EDITION

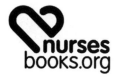

nurses
books.org

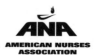

**AMERICAN NURSES
ASSOCIATION**

American Nurses Association
Silver Spring, Maryland
2010

Library of Congress Cataloging-in-Publication data

American Nurses Association.
 Nursing : scope and standards of practice. — 2nd ed.
  p. ; cm.
 Includes bibliographical references and index.
 ISBN-13: 978-1-55810-282-8 (pbk.)
 ISBN-10: 1-55810-282-5 (pbk.)
 1. Nursing—Standards—United States. I. Title.
 [DNLM: 1. Nursing—standards—United States—Practice Guideline.   2. Clinical Competence—
 standards—United States—Practice Guideline.   WY 16]
 RT85.5.A47 2010
 610.7302′1873—dc22   2010028581

The American Nurses Association (ANA) is a national professional association. This ANA publication—*Nursing: Scope and Standards of Practice, Second Edition*—reflects the thinking of the nursing profession on various issues and should be reviewed in conjunction with state board of nursing policies and practices. State law, rules, and regulations govern the practice of nursing, while *Nursing: Scope and Standards of Practice, Second Edition* guides nurses in the application of their professional skills and responsibilities. For more about the American Nurses, see page xii.

Published by Nursesbooks.org
The Publishing Program of ANA
www.Nursesbooks.org/

American Nurses Association
8515 Georgia Avenue, Suite 400
Silver Spring, MD 20910-3492
1-800-274-4ANA
www.NursingWorld.org

DESIGN: David Fox, AURAS Design, Silver Spring, Maryland
TYPESETTING: House of Equations, Arden, North Carolina
PRINTING: McArdle Printing, Upper Marlboro, Maryland
EDITORIAL SERVICES: Steve A. Jent, Denton, TX (copyediting); Grammarians, Inc., Washington, DC: Kelly Saxton (proofreading); Eric Wurzbacher, Silver Spring, MD (indexing).

ISBN-13: 978-1-55810-282-8   SAN: 851-3481   30M   08/2010

First printing: August 2010

Contents

Contributors

Nursing: Scope and Standards of Practice, Second Edition is the product of significant thought work by many registered nurses and a four-step review process involving those listed below. The document originated from the decisions garnered during a significant number of telephone conference calls and electronic mail communications of the diverse workgroup members, then followed by an extensive public comment period. The review process included two evaluations by the Committee on Nursing Practice Standards and Guidelines of ANA's Congress on Nursing Practice and Economics, review and approval by the entire Congress on Nursing Practice and Economics, and finally, review and approval by the American Nurses Association Board of Directors in May 2010. The list of endorsing organizations that completes this section reflects the broad acceptance of this resource within the profession.

Nursing Scope and Standards Workgroup, 2009–2010

Ann O'Sullivan, MSN, RN, NE-BC, CNE – Chair
    Julia Rose Barcott, RN
    Nancy Bonalumi, MS, RN, CEN, FAEN
    Susan B. Collins, FNP-BC, AHN-BC
    Louise Darling, BSN, RNC, IBCLC
    Gwen A. Davis, MN, RN, CDE
    Melanie Duffy, MSN, RN, CCRN, CCNS
    Diane Earl, RN
    Janice Cooke Feigenbaum, PhD, RN
    Jacqueline Fournier, APRN, BC
    Michael J. Kremer, PhD, CRNA, FAAN

Kathleen A.V. Lavery, MS, CNM
Beth Martin, MSN, RN, CCNS, ACNP-BC, ACHP
Deborah Maust Martin, MSN, RN, MBA, NE-BC, FACHE
Mary-Anne Ponti, MSN, MBA, RN, CNAA-BC
Harry F. Smith, CDR, NC, USN
Juan Carlos Soto, EdD, MSN, RN
Cindy Diamond Zolnierek, MSN, RN

(For more about the workgroup, go to this book's record at
www.Nursesbooks.org.)

ANA Staff, 2009–2010

Carol J. Bickford, PhD, RN-BC	Content editor
Katherine C. Brewer, MSN, RN	Content editor
Maureen E. Cones, Esq.	Legal counsel
Yvonne Humes, MSA	Project coordinator
Eric Wurzbacher	Project editor

Committee on Nursing Practice Standards and Guidelines. 2009–2010

Tresha L. Lucas, MSN, RN, CNAA-BC – Chair
Rosemary Pais Brown, MSN, RN
Julia A. Dangel, MSN, RN
Judith Harris, EdD, ARNP
Richard Henker, PhD, RN, CRNA
Wanda Lewis, DHA, RN, CCRN
Sandi McDermott, RN, MSN, NEA-BC
Margaret Nelson, MS, RN
Elizabeth Libby Thomas, Med, RN, NCSN, FNASN

Congress on Nursing Practice and Economics, 2008–2010

CHAIR
Kathleen M. White, PhD, RN, CNAA-BC

VICE-CHAIR
Ann M. O'Sullivan, RN, MSN, NE-BC, CNE

MEMBERS

Susan A. Albrecht, PhD, RN, FAAN

Mary L. Behrens, RN, MSN, FNP-C

Carolyn Baird, MBA, MEd, RN-BC, CARN-AP, CCDP-D-Diplomate
International Nurses Society on Addictions

Carola M. Bruflat, RNC, MSN, WHNP-BC/FNP-BC
Association of Women's Health, Obstetrics and Neonatal Nurses

Garry Brydges, MSN, ACNP-BS, CRNA

Stephanie Davis Burnett, MSN, RN, ACNSpBC, CRRN
Association of Rehabilitation Nurses

Mary Eileen Callan, MS, RN, FNP-BC

Myra C. Carmon, EdD, CPNP, RN

Robin Chard, PhD, RN, CNOR
Association of periOperative Registered Nurses

Thomas Coe, RN, PhD, NEA-BC, FACHE

John F. Dixon, MSN, RN, NE-BC
American Association of Critical-Care Nurses

William R. Donovan, MA, RN

Merilyn Douglass, ARNP, MSN

Bette M. Ferree, RN, MSN, FNP-BC

Susan Foster, MSN, RN, FNP-BC

Lisa A. Gorski, MS, HHCNS-BC, CRNI, FAAN
Infusion Nurses Society

Janet Y. Harris, RN, MSN, CNAA-BC

Kimberly A. Hickey, MSN, APRN-BC

Debra Hobbins, MSN, APRN

Patricia L. Holloman, BSN, RN, CNOR

Patricia K. Howard, PhD, RN, CEN
Emergency Nurses Association

Sally Burrows-Hudson, MS, RN, CNN
American Nephrology Nurses Association

Bette K. Idemoto, PhD, RN, CCRN, CS

Sandra Gracia Jones, PhD, ARNP, CS-C, ACRN, FAAN

Beverly Jorgenson, RNC, MSN, NNP

David M. Keepnews, PhD, JD, RN, FAAN

Patricia L. Keller, MSN, RN, NE-BC

Patrick E. Kenny, EdD, RN-BC, ACRN, APRN-PMH, NE-C
Association of Nurses in AIDS Care

Linda Riazi-Kermani, BSN, RN, CEN

Robin R. Potter-Kimball, RN, MS, CNS-BC

Jane Kirschling, DNS, RN
American Association of Colleges of Nursing

Pamela A. Kulbok, DNSc, RN, PhCNS-BC

Kathleen G. Lawrence, MSN, RN, CWOCN
Wound Ostomy Continence Nurses Society

Carla A. B. Lee, PhD, ARNP-BC, CNAA, FAAN

Lori Lioce, MSN, FNP-BC

Jennifer H. Matthews, PhD, ACNS-BC

Sara A. McCumber, RN, CNP, CNS

Peter T. Mitchell, MSN, RN, CNP, APRN-BC

Karen Leone-Natale, BSN, RN

Pamela Sue Neal, MSN-NA, RN, FNP, APRN-BC

Catherine E. Neuman, MSN, RN, NEA-BC

Linda L. Olson, PhD, RN, NEA-BC

Jackie R. Pfeifer, RN, MSN, CCRN-CSC, CCNS

Theresa A. Posani, MS, RN, CNS, APRN-BC, CCRN, CNE

Elizabeth Poster, PhD, RN, FAAN

Susan E. Reinarz, RN, MSN, NNP-BC
National Association of Neonatal Nurses

Cheryl-Ann Resha, EdD, MSN, RN
National Association of School Nurses

Patricia Schlosser, BSN, RN

Cheryl K. Schmidt, PhD, RN, CNE, ANEF

Sue Sendelbach, PhD, RN, CCNS
National Association of Clinical Nurse Specialists

Nancy Shirley, PhD, RN

Joanna Sikkema, MSN, ARNP, FAHA
Preventive Cardiovascular Nurses Association

Elaine L. Smith, MSN, MBA, RN, CNAA
National Nursing Staff Development Organization

Karen J. Stanley, RN, MSN, AOCN, FAAN
Oncology Nursing Society

Thomas E. Stenvig, RN, PhD, MPH, CNAA

Mary Mason Wyckoff, PhD, MSN, ACNP-BC, FNP-BC, NNP, CCNS, CCRN

About the American Nurses Association

The American Nurses Association (ANA) is the only full-service professional organization representing the interests of the nation's 3.1 million registered nurses through its constituent member nurses associations, its organizational affiliates, and the Center for American Nurses. The ANA advances the nursing profession by fostering high standards of nursing practice, promoting the rights of nurses in the workplace, projecting a positive and realistic view of nursing, and by lobbying the Congress and regulatory agencies on health care issues affecting nurses and the public.

About Nursesbooks.org,
The Publishing Program of ANA

Nursesbooks.org publishes books on ANA core issues and programs, including ethics, leadership, quality, specialty practice, advanced practice, and the profession's enduring legacy. Best known for the foundational documents of the profession on nursing ethics, scope and standards of practice, and social policy, Nursesbooks.org is the publisher for the professional, career-oriented nurse, reaching and serving nurse educators, administrators, managers, and researchers as well as staff nurses in the course of their professional development.

Endorsing Organizations

The following organizations have formally endorsed *Nursing: Scope and Standards of Practice, Second Edition* as of August 18, 2010. Names of other endorsing organizations will be added in an updated version of this list at http://www.nursingworld.org/MainMenuCategories/ThePracticeofProfessionalNursing/NursingStandards.aspx

Academy of Medical-Surgical Nurses

Academy of Neonatal Nursing

Air and Surface Transport Nurses

American Academy of Ambulatory Care Nursing

American Association of Colleges of Nursing

American Association of Critical-Care Nurses

American Association of Heart Failure Nurses

American Association of Legal Nurse Consultants

American Association of Neuroscience Nurses

American Association of Nurse Anesthetists

American College of Nurse-Midwives

American College of Nurse Practitioners

American Holistic Nurses Association

American Nephrology Nurses' Association

American Pediatric Surgical Nurses Association

American Psychiatric Nurses Association

American Society for Parenteral and Enteral Nutrition, including the Nutrition Support Nurse Practice Section

American Society of Plastic Surgical Nursing

Association of Nurses in AIDS Care

Association of Pediatric Hematology/Oncology Nurses

Association of periOperative Registered Nurses

Association of Rehabilitation Nurses

Association of Women's Health, Obstetric and Neonatal Nurses

Center for American Nurses and Institute for Nursing Research and Education

Dermatology Nurses' Association, including the Nurse Practitioner Society of the Dermatology Nurses' Association

Emergency Nurses Association

Infusion Nurses Society

International Association of Forensic Nurses

International Nurses Society on Addictions

National Association of Clinical Nurse Specialists

National Association of Neonatal Nurses

National Association of Orthopaedic Nurses

National Association of Pediatric Nurse Practitioners

National Association of School Nurses

National Gerontological Nursing Association

National Nursing Staff Development Organization

National Student Nurses' Association, Inc.

Oncology Nursing Society

Pediatric Endocrinology Nursing Society

Preventive Cardiovascular Nurses Association

Society of Gastroenterology Nurses and Associates

Society of Otorhinolaryngology and Head-Neck Nurses

Society of Pediatric Nurses

Society of Trauma Nurses

Society of Urologic Nurses and Associates

Wound, Ostomy and Continence Nurses Society

Overview of the Content

Foundational Documents of Professional Nursing

Registered nurses practicing in the United States have three professional resources that inform their thinking and decision-making and guide their practice. First, *Code of Ethics for Nurses with Interpretive Statements* (ANA, 2001) lists the nine succinct provisions that establish the ethical framework for registered nurses across all roles, levels, and settings. Second, *Nursing's Social Policy Statement: The Essence of the Profession* (ANA, 2010) conceptualizes nursing practice, describes the social context of nursing, and provides the definition of nursing.

Nursing: Scope and Standards of Practice, Second Edition, outlines the expectations of the professional role of the registered nurse. It states the Scope of Practice and presents the Standards of Professional Nursing Practice and their accompanying competencies.

Additional Content

For a better appreciation of the history and context related to *Nursing: Scope and Standards of Practice, Second Edition*, readers will find the additional content of the four appendixes useful:

- Appendix A. ANA's Principles of Environmental Health for Nursing
  Practice

- Appendix B. Professional Role Competence: ANA Position Statement

- Appendix C. The Development of Foundational Nursing Documents and Professional Nursing

- Appendix D. Nursing: Scope and Standards of Practice (2004)

Audience for This Publication

Registered nurses in every role and setting constitute the primary audience of this professional resource. Legislators, regulators, legal counsel, and the judiciary system will also want to reference it. Agencies, organizations, nurse administrators, and interprofessional colleagues will find this an invaluable reference. In addition, the people, families, communities, and populations using healthcare and nursing services can use this document to better understand what constitutes nursing and who its members are: registered nurses and advanced practice registered nurses

Scope of
Nursing Practice

Definition of Nursing

Nursing's Social Policy Statement: The Essence of the Profession (ANA, 2010, p. 3) builds on previous work and provides the following contemporary definition of nursing:

> *Nursing is the protection, promotion, and optimization of health and abilities, prevention of illness and injury, alleviation of suffering through the diagnosis and treatment of human response, and advocacy in the care of individuals, families, communities, and populations.*

This definition serves as the foundation for the following expanded description of the Scope of Nursing Practice and the Standards of Professional Nursing Practice.

Professional Nursing's Scope and Standards of Practice

A professional nursing organization has a responsibility to its members and to the public it serves to develop the scope and standards of its profession's practice. As the professional organization for all registered nurses, the American Nurses Association (ANA) has assumed the responsibility for developing the scope and standards that apply to the practice of all professional nurses and serve as a template for nursing specialty practice. Standards do, however, belong to the profession and, thus, require broad input into their development and revision. *Nursing: Scope and Standards of Practice, Second Edition,* describes a competent level of nursing practice and professional performance common to all registered nurses.

Description of the Scope of Nursing Practice

The scope of practice statement describes the "who," "what," "where," "when," "why," and "how" of nursing practice. Each of these questions must be answered to provide a complete picture of the dynamic and complex practice of nursing and its evolving boundaries and membership. The profession of nursing has one scope of practice that encompasses the full range of nursing practice, pertinent to general and specialty practice. The depth and breadth in which individual registered nurses engage in the total scope of nursing practice are dependent on their education, experience, role, and the population served.

Development and Function of Nursing Standards

The Standards of Professional Nursing Practice are authoritative statements of the duties that all registered nurses, regardless of role, population, or specialty, are expected to perform competently. The standards published herein may serve as evidence of the standard of care, with the understanding that application of the standards depends on context. The standards are subject to change with the dynamics of the nursing profession, as new patterns of professional practice are developed and accepted by the nursing profession and the public. In addition, specific conditions and clinical circumstances may also affect the application of the standards at a given time, e.g., during a natural disaster. The standards are subject to formal, periodic review and revision.

The Function of Competencies in Standards

The competencies that accompany each standard may be evidence of compliance with the corresponding standard. The list of competencies is not exhaustive. Whether a particular standard or competency applies depends upon the circumstances. For example, a nurse providing treatment to an unconscious, critical patient who presented to the hospital by ambulance without family has a duty to collect comprehensive data pertinent to the patient's health (Standard 1. Assessment). However, under the attendant circumstances, that nurse may not be expected to assess family dynamics and impact on the patient's health and wellness (Assessment Competency). In the same circumstance, Standard 5B. Health Teaching and Health Promotion may not apply at all.

The Nursing Process

The *nursing process* is often conceptualized as the integration of singular actions of assessment, diagnosis, and identification of outcomes, planning, implementation, and finally, evaluation. The nursing process in practice is not linear as often conceptualized, with a feedback loop from evaluation to assessment. Rather, it relies heavily on the bi-directional feedback loops from each component, as illustrated in Figure 1.

The Standards of Practice coincide with the steps of the nursing process to represent the directive nature of the standards as the professional nurse completes each component of the nursing process. Similarly, the Standards of Professional Performance relate to how the professional nurse adheres to the Standards of Practice, completes the nursing process, and addresses other nursing practice issues and concerns (ANA, 2010). Five tenets characterize contemporary nursing practice (see next two pages).

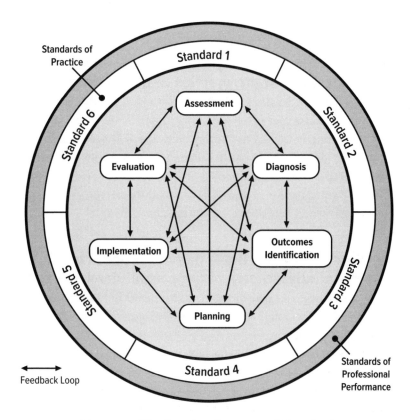

FIGURE 1. The Nursing Process and Standards of Professional Nursing Practice

Tenets Characteristic of Nursing Practice.

1. Nursing practice is individualized.

Nursing practice respects diversity and is individualized to meet the unique needs of the healthcare consumer or situation. *Healthcare consumer* is defined to be the patient, person, client, family, group, community, or population who is the focus of attention and to whom the registered nurse is providing services as sanctioned by the state regulatory bodies.

2. Nurses coordinate care by establishing partnerships.

The registered nurse establishes partnerships with persons, families, support systems, and other providers, utilizing in-person and electronic communications, to reach a shared goal of delivering health care. Health care is defined as the attempt "to address the health needs of the patient and the public" (ANA, 2001, p. 10). Collaborative interprofessional team planning is based on recognition of each discipline's value and contributions, mutual trust, respect, open discussion, and shared decision-making.

3. Caring is central to the practice of the registered nurse.

Professional nursing promotes healing and health in a way that builds a relationship between nurse and patient (Watson, 1999, 2008). "Caring is a conscious judgment that manifests itself in concrete acts, interpersonally, verbally, and nonverbally" (Gallagher-Lepak & Kubsch, 2009, p. 171). While caring for individuals, families, and populations is the key focus of nursing, the nurse additionally promotes self-care as well as care of the environment and society (Hagerty, Lynch-Sauer, Patusky, & Bouwseman, 1993).

4. Registered nurses use the nursing process to plan and provide individualized care to their healthcare consumers.

Nurses use theoretical and evidence-based knowledge of human experiences and responses to collaborate with healthcare consumers to assess, diagnose, identify outcomes, plan, implement, and evaluate care. Nursing interventions are intended to produce beneficial effects, contribute to quality outcomes, and above all, do no harm. Nurses evaluate the effectiveness of their care in relation to identified outcomes and use evidence-based practice to improve care (ANA,

2010). Critical thinking underlies each step of the nursing process, problem-solving, and decision-making. The nursing process is cyclical and dynamic, interpersonal and collaborative, and universally applicable.

5. A strong link exists between the professional work environment and the registered nurse's ability to provide quality health care and achieve optimal outcomes.

Professional nurses have an ethical obligation to maintain and improve health-care practice environments conducive to the provision of quality health care (ANA, 2001). Extensive studies have demonstrated the relationship between effective nursing practice and the presence of a healthy work environment. Mounting evidence demonstrates that negative, demoralizing, and unsafe conditions in the workplace (unhealthy work environments) contribute to medical errors, ineffective delivery of care, and conflict and stress among health professionals.

Healthy Work Environments for Nursing Practice

ANA supports the following models of healthy work environment design:

AMERICAN ASSOCIATION OF CRITICAL-CARE NURSES

The American Association of Critical-Care Nurses has identified six standards for establishing and maintaining healthy work environments (AACN, 2005):

- *Skilled Communication*
  Nurses must be as proficient in communication skills as they are in clinical skills.

- *True Collaboration*
  Nurses must be relentless in pursuing and fostering a sense of team and partnership across all disciplines.

- *Effective Decision-making*
  Nurses are seen as valued and committed partners in making policy, directing and evaluating clinical care, and leading organizational operations.

- *Appropriate Staffing*
  Staffing must ensure the effective match between healthcare consumer needs and nurse competencies.

- *Meaningful Recognition*
  Nurses must be recognized and must recognize others for the value each brings to the work of the organization.

- *Authentic Leadership*
  Nurse leaders must fully embrace the imperative of a healthy work environment, authentically live it, and engage others in achieving it.

MAGNET RECOGNITION PROGRAM

The Magnet Recognition Program® addresses the professional work environment, requiring that Magnet®-designated facilities adhere to the following model components (ANCC, 2008):

- *Transformational Leadership*
  The transformational leader leads people where they need to be in order to meet the demands of the future.

- *Structural Empowerment*
  Structures and processes developed by influential leadership provide an innovative practice environment in which strong professional practice flourishes and the mission, vision, and values come to life to achieve the outcomes believed to be important for the organization.

- *Exemplary Professional Practice*
  This demonstrates what professional nursing practice can achieve.

- *New Knowledge, Innovation, and Improvements*
  Organizations have an ethical and professional responsibility to contribute to healthcare delivery, the organization, and the profession.

- *Empirical Quality Results*
  Organizations are in a unique position to become pioneers of the future and to demonstrate solutions to numerous problems inherent in today's healthcare systems. Beyond the "What" and "How," organizations must ask themselves what difference these efforts have made

INSTITUTE OF MEDICINE

The Institute of Medicine has also reported that safety and quality problems occur when dedicated health professionals work in systems that neither support them nor prepare them to achieve optimal patient care outcomes (IOM, 2004). Such rapid changes as reimbursement modification and cost containment efforts, new healthcare technologies, and changes in the health-care workforce have influenced the work and work environment of nurses. Accordingly, concentration on key aspects of the work environment—people, physical surroundings, and tools—can enhance healthcare working conditions and improve patient safety. These include:

- Transformational leadership and evidence-based management

- Maximizing workforce capability

- Creating and sustaining a culture of safety and research

- Work space design and redesign to prevent and mitigate errors

- Effective use of telecommunications and biomedical device interoperability

Model of Professional Nursing Practice Regulation

In 2006 the Model of Professional Nursing Practice Regulation (see Figure 2) emerged from ANA work and informed the discussions of specialty nursing and advanced practice registered nurse practice.

The lowest level in the model represents the responsibility of the professional and specialty nursing organizations to their members and the public to define the scope and standards of practice for nursing.

The next level up the pyramid represents the regulation provided by the nurse practice acts and the rules and regulations in the pertinent licensing juris-

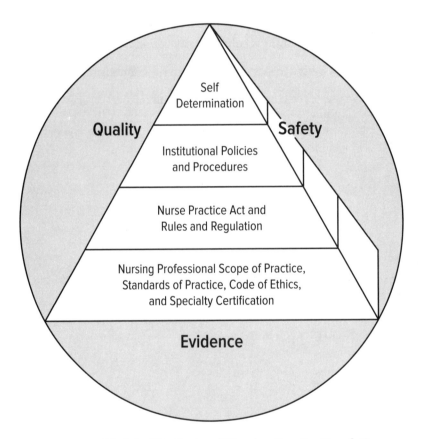

FIGURE 2. Model of Professional Nursing Practice Regulation (Styles et al., 2008).

dictions. Institutional policies and procedures provide further considerations in the regulation of nursing practice for the registered nurse and advanced practice registered nurse.

Note that the highest level is that of self determination by the nurse after consideration of all the other levels of input about professional nursing practice regulation. The outcome is safe, quality, and evidence-based practice.

Standards of Professional Nursing Practice

The Standards of Professional Nursing Practice content consists of the Standards of Practice and the Standards of Professional Performance.

Standards of Practice

The Standards of Practice describe a competent level of nursing care as demonstrated by the critical thinking model known as the nursing process. The nursing process includes the components of assessment, diagnosis, outcomes identification, planning, implementation, and evaluation. Accordingly, the nursing process encompasses significant actions taken by registered nurses and forms the foundation of the nurse's decision-making.

STANDARD 1. ASSESSMENT

The registered nurse collects comprehensive data pertinent to the healthcare consumer's health and/or the situation.

STANDARD 2. DIAGNOSIS

The registered nurse analyzes the assessment data to determine the diagnoses or the issues.

STANDARD 3. OUTCOMES IDENTIFICATION

The registered nurse identifies expected outcomes for a plan individualized to the healthcare consumer or the situation.

STANDARD 4. PLANNING

The registered nurse develops a plan that prescribes strategies and alternatives to attain expected outcomes.

STANDARD 5. IMPLEMENTATION
The registered nurse implements the identified plan.

STANDARD 5A. COORDINATION OF CARE
The registered nurse coordinates care delivery.

STANDARD 5B. HEALTH TEACHING AND HEALTH PROMOTION
The registered nurse employs strategies to promote health and a safe environment.

STANDARD 5C. CONSULTATION
The graduate-level prepared specialty nurse or advanced practice registered nurse provides consultation to influence the identified plan, enhance the abilities of others, and effect change.

STANDARD 5D. PRESCRIPTIVE AUTHORITY AND TREATMENT
The advanced practice registered nurse uses prescriptive authority, procedures, referrals, treatments, and therapies in accordance with state and federal laws and regulations.

STANDARD 6. EVALUATION
The registered nurse evaluates progress toward attainment of outcomes.

Standards of Professional Performance
The Standards of Professional Performance describe a competent level of behavior in the professional role, including activities related to ethics, education, evidence-based practice and research, quality of practice, communication, leadership, collaboration, professional practice evaluation, resource utilization, and environmental health. All registered nurses are expected to engage in professional role activities, including leadership, appropriate to their education and position. Registered nurses are accountable for their professional actions to themselves, their healthcare consumers, their peers, and ultimately to society.

STANDARD 7. ETHICS
The registered nurse practices ethically.

STANDARD 8. EDUCATION
The registered nurse attains knowledge and competence that reflects current nursing practice.

STANDARD 9. EVIDENCE-BASED PRACTICE AND RESEARCH
The registered nurse integrates evidence and research findings into practice.

STANDARD 10. QUALITY OF PRACTICE
The registered nurse contributes to quality nursing practice.

STANDARD 11. COMMUNICATION
The registered nurse communicates effectively in all areas of practice.

STANDARD 12. LEADERSHIP
The registered nurse demonstrates leadership in the professional practice setting and the profession.

STANDARD 13. COLLABORATION
The registered nurse collaborates with healthcare consumer, family, and others in the conduct of nursing practice.

STANDARD 14. PROFESSIONAL PRACTICE EVALUATION
The registered nurse evaluates her or his own nursing practice in relation to professional practice standards and guidelines, relevant statutes, rules, and regulations.

STANDARD 15. RESOURCE UTILIZATION
The registered nurse utilizes appropriate resources to plan and provide nursing services that are safe, effective, and financially responsible.

STANDARD 16. ENVIRONMENTAL HEALTH
The registered nurse practices in an environmentally safe and healthy manner.

Professional Competence in Nursing Practice

The public has a right to expect registered nurses to demonstrate professional competence throughout their careers. The registered nurse is individually responsible and accountable for maintaining professional competence. It is the nursing profession's responsibility to shape and guide any process for assuring nurse competence. Regulatory agencies define minimal standards of competency to protect the public. The employer is responsible and accountable to provide a practice environment conducive to competent practice. Assurance of competence is the shared responsibility of the profession, individual nurses, professional organizations, credentialing and certification entities, regulatory agencies, employers, and other key stakeholders (ANA, 2008).

ANA believes that in the practice of nursing competence can be defined, measured, and evaluated. No single evaluation method or tool can guarantee competence. Competence is situational and dynamic; it is both an outcome and an ongoing process. Context determines what competencies are necessary.

Definitions and Concepts Related to Competence

A number of terms are central to the discussion of competence:

- An individual who demonstrates "competence" is performing at an expected level.

- A *competency* is an expected level of performance that integrates knowledge, skills, abilities, and judgment.

- The integration of knowledge, skills, abilities, and judgment occurs in formal, informal, and reflective learning experiences.

- Knowledge encompasses thinking, understanding of science and humanities, professional standards of practice, and insights gained from context, practical experiences, personal capabilities, and leadership performance.

- Skills include psychomotor, communication, interpersonal, and diagnostic skills.

- Ability is the capacity to act effectively. It requires listening, integrity, knowledge of one's strengths and weaknesses, positive self-regard, emotional intelligence, and openness to feedback.

- Judgment includes critical thinking, problem solving, ethical reasoning, and decision-making.

- *Formal learning* most often occurs in structured, academic, and professional development practice environments, while informal learning can be described as experiential insights gained in work, community, home, and other settings.

- *Reflective learning* represents the recurrent thoughtful personal self-assessment, analysis, and synthesis of strengths and opportunities for improvement. Such insights should lead to the creation of a specific plan for professional development and may become part of one's professional portfolio (ANA, 2008).

Competence and Competency in Nursing Practice

Competent registered nurses can be influenced by the nature of the situation, which includes consideration of the setting, resources, and the person. Situations can either enhance or detract from the nurse's ability to perform. The registered nurse influences factors that facilitate and enhance competent practice. Similarly, the nurse seeks to deal with barriers that constrain competent practice. The expected level of performance reflects variability depending upon context and the selected competence framework or model.

The ability to perform at the expected level requires a process of lifelong learning. Registered nurses must continually reassess their competencies and identify needs for additional knowledge, skills, personal growth, and integrative learning experiences.

Evaluating Competence

"Competence in nursing practice must be evaluated by the individual nurse (self-assessment), nurse peers, and nurses in the roles of supervisor, coach, mentor, or preceptor. In addition, other aspects of nursing performance may be evaluated by professional colleagues and patients.

Competence can be evaluated by using tools that capture objective and subjective data about the individual's knowledge base and actual performance and are appropriate for the specific situation and the desired outcome of the competence evaluation . . . However, no single evaluation tool or method can guarantee competence" (ANA, 2008, p. 6).

Professional Registered Nurses Today

Statistical Snapshot

In 2008, there were an estimated 3 million registered nurses (RNs) in the United States, of which 2.6 million are currently employed. The majority of registered nurses initially entered nursing with an associate degree; however, the percentage of nurses entering practice with a bachelor's degree or higher has increased steadily. Most registered nurses work in hospitals (62%) and identify themselves as "staff nurses" (66%).

In addition to hospitals, nurses report working in ambulatory care (10%), public/community health (7.8%), home health (6.4%), nursing home/extended care (5.3%), academic education (3.8%), and other areas, including insurance, benefits, and utilization review (3.9%). Public/community health includes school and occupational health settings, and ambulatory care includes medical and physician practices, health centers and clinics, and other types of non-hospital clinic settings.

About 9% of nurses identify themselves as one of the four recognized advanced practice registered nurse roles, and other identified roles include management, patient coordinator, instructor, patient educator, and researcher. (U.S. Dept. of Labor, 2010; U.S. DHHS, 2010)

Licensure and Education of Registered Nurses

The registered nurse is licensed and authorized by a state, commonwealth, or territory to practice nursing. Professional licensure of the healthcare professions is established by each jurisdiction to protect the public safety and authorize the practice of the profession. Because of this, the requirements for RN licensure and advanced practice nursing vary widely.

The registered nurse is educationally prepared for competent practice at the beginning level upon graduation from an accredited school of nursing and qualified by national examination for RN licensure. ANA has consistently affirmed the baccalaureate degree in nursing as the preferred educational preparation for entry into nursing practice.

The registered nurse is educated in the art and science of nursing, with the goal of helping individuals and groups attain, maintain, and restore health whenever possible. Experienced nurses may become proficient in one or more practice areas or roles. These nurses may concentrate on healthcare consumer care in clinical nursing practice specialties. Others influence nursing and support the direct care rendered to healthcare consumers by those professional nurses in clinical practice. Credentialing is one form of acknowledging such specialized knowledge and experience. Credentialing organizations may mandate specific nursing educational requirements, as well as timely demonstrations of knowledge and experience in specialty practice.

Registered nurses may pursue advanced academic studies to prepare for specialization in practice. Educational requirements vary by specialty and educational program. New models for educational preparation are evolving in response to the changing healthcare, education, and regulatory practice environments.

Roots of Professional Nursing

Nursing has evolved into a profession with a distinct body of knowledge, university-based education, specialized practice, standards of practice, a social contract (ANA, 2010), and an ethical code (ANA, 2001). With this grounding, registered nurses and their profession are concerned with the availability and accessibility of nursing care to healthcare consumers, families, communities, and populations, and seek to ensure the integrity of nursing practice in all current and future healthcare systems. This professional evolution is described in the following pages.

Nursing Research and Evidence-Based Practice

Contemporary nursing practice has its historical roots in the poorhouses, the battlefields, and the industrial revolutions in nineteenth-century Europe and America. Initially nurses trained in hospital-based nursing schools and were employed mainly providing private care to patients in their homes. Florence Nightingale provided a foundation for nursing and the basis for autonomous nursing practice as distinct from medicine. Nightingale also is credited with identifying the importance of collecting empirical evidence, the underpinning of nursing's current emphasis on evidence-based practice, "What you want are facts, not opinions . . . The most important practical lesson that can be given to nurses is to teach them what to observe—how to observe—what symptoms indicate improvement—which are of none—which are the evidence of neglect—and what kind of neglect." (Nightingale, 1859, p. 105)

Although Nightingale recommended clinical nursing research in the mid-1800s, nurses did not follow her advice for over 100 years. Nursing research was able to flourish only as nurses received advanced educational preparation.

In the early 1900s nurses received their advanced degrees in nursing education, and thus nursing research was limited to studies of nurses and nursing education. However, case studies on nursing interventions were conducted in the 1920s and 1930s and the results published in the *American Journal of Nursing*.

In the 1950s, interest in nursing care studies began to rise. In 1952, the first issue of *Nursing Research* was published. In the 1960s, nursing studies began to explore theoretical and conceptual frameworks as a basis for practice. By the 1970s, more doctorally prepared nurses were conducting research, especially studies related to practice and the improvement of patient care. By the 1980s, there were greater numbers of qualified nurse researchers than ever before, and more computers available for collection and analysis of data. In 1985, the National Center for Nursing Research was established within the National Institutes of Health, putting nursing research into the mainstream of health research (Grant and Massey, 1999).

In the last half of the twentieth century, nurse researchers (1950s) and nurse theorists (1960s and 1970s) greatly contributed to the expanding body of nursing knowledge with their studies of nursing practice and the development of nursing models and theories. These conceptual models and theories borrow from other disciplines such as sociology, psychology, biology, and physics.

For example, the work of Neuman and King makes extensive use of systems theory. There is also Levine's conservation model, Roger's science of unitary human beings, Roy's adaptation model, Orem's self-care model, Peplau's interpersonal relations model, and Watson's theory of caring. The 1980s brought revisions to these theories, as well as additional theories developed by nursing leaders, such as Johnson, Parse, and Leininger, that added to the theoretical basis of nursing (George, 2002). In the 1990s, research tested and expanded these theories, which in turn continued to define and elaborate the discipline of nursing.

Evidence-based practice (EBP) is a scholarly and systematic problem-solving paradigm that results in the delivery of high-quality health care. In order to make the best clinical decisions using EBP, external evidence from research is blended with internal evidence (i.e., practice-generated data), clinical expertise, and healthcare consumer values and preferences to achieve the best outcomes for individuals, groups, populations, and healthcare systems.

Nursing's embrace of EBP is part of a larger call to integrate it into the entire spectrum of healthcare disciplines and professions. The Institute of Medicine (IOM) developed a vision for clinical education in the health professions that is centered on a commitment to meeting patient needs (IOM, 2003). This report stresses that all health disciplines must embrace evidence-based practice, quality improvement, and informatics in delivering healthcare consumer-centered care, and that their education should reflect and teach them to value those competencies. Interprofessional team collaboration is necessary to achieve quality outcomes for the improvement of health care.

Nursing research and EBP contribute to the body of knowledge and enhance outcomes. As a profession, nursing continually evaluates and applies nursing research findings. Evaluation of outcomes is a critical step in EBP. New knowledge is translated to healthcare consumer care to promote effective and efficient care and improved outcomes. It is then disseminated to decrease practice variations, improve outcomes, and create standards of excellence for care and policies. In addition, nurses ensure that changes in practice are based on current evidence; they should have expert resources in their practice environment and seek out those resources to assist them with specific steps in EBP.

The complex dynamics of health care, and demands for healthcare reform, will challenge the profession to quantify and qualify the value of nursing and nursing care. In alignment with the current edition of *Nursing's Social Policy Statement* (ANA, 2010) and this publication, the nursing profession continually examines nursing practice. An example is the study of unit-based nurse staffing levels, and demonstrating through evidence that safe staffing is imperative to quality patient care. This includes ongoing systematic evaluation of the impact of staffing and staffing effectiveness on patient outcomes.

Nursing's foundation as a profession took shape in the nineteenth century under Florence Nightingale, most notably with her work to provide quality nursing care for British soldiers during the Crimean War. But Nightingale also encouraged nurses to care for people beyond the sick bed, and to improve the health and safety of communities to promote wellness and prevent death (Nightingale, 1859). In the succeeding 150 years, nursing has expanded to almost every theater of health care.

Specialty Practice in Nursing

Nursing first expanded into public health interventions on behalf of at-risk communities and vulnerable populations. In 1893, Lillian Wald pioneered public health nursing at the Henry Street Settlement House in New York City. In 1899, Teacher's College at Columbia University offered the first university program for graduate nurses to specialize in public health nursing (Stewart, 1948). An editorial in the *American Journal of Nursing* in 1911 pointed out the urgent demand for nurses who could teach others and who could organize a whole community.

In the mid-twentieth century and beyond, advances in medical treatment and healthcare technology led to the evolution of other nursing specialties. Specialized education, training, and certification ensued in both traditional and newer areas of clinical practice, including medical-surgical nursing, pediatrics, anesthesia, midwifery, emergency care, mental health, public health, critical care, neonatal care, and primary care.

The continuation of the profession depends on the education of nurses, appropriate organization of nursing services, continued expansion of nursing knowledge, and the development and adoption of policies. Such initiatives demand that registered nurses be adequately prepared for these nursing specialties. Some specialties reflect the intersection of nursing's body of knowledge and that of another profession or discipline, directly influence nursing practice, and support the delivery of direct care rendered by registered nurses to healthcare consumers. Specialty nurses collaborate, consult, and serve as a liaison, bridging the role of the professional registered nurse with that of other professionals, and subsequently help to delineate nursing's role in society.

Registered nurses in specialty practice represent the full spectrum from novice to expert. Many nurses with an advanced graduate nursing education practice in specialties, such as informatics, public health, education, or administration, that are essential to advancing the public health but do not focus on direct care to individuals. Therefore, their practice does not require regulatory recognition beyond the Registered Nurse license granted by state boards of nursing.

Similarly, advanced practice registered nurses acquire specialized knowledge and skills through graduate-level education in their selected specialty areas. Competencies in individual specialty areas of practice are defined by separate specialty scope and standards documents, authored by specialty nursing associations. Many specialty nursing organizations recognize individual expertise through national certification in the specialty (see pages 92–94).

Advanced Practice Registered Nurse Roles

Another evolution of nursing practice was the development of educational programs to prepare nurses for advanced practice in direct care roles. These Advanced Practice Registered Nurse (APRN) roles include Certified Registered Nurse Anesthetists (CRNAs), Certified Nurse-Midwives (CNMs), Clinical

Nurse Specialists (CNSs), and Certified Nurse Practitioners (CNPs). Each has a unique history and context, but shares a focus on direct care to individual healthcare consumers.

Advanced Practice Registered Nurse is a regulatory title and includes the four roles listed above. The core competencies for education and the scope of practice are defined by the professional associations. State law and regulation further define criteria for licensure for the designated scopes of practice. The need to ensure healthcare consumer safety and access to APRNs by aligning education, accreditation, licensure, and certification is shown in *Consensus Model for APRN Regulation: Licensure, Accreditation, Certification, and Education* (APRN JDG, 2008).

In addition to the licensure, accreditation, certification, and education requirements for advanced practice registered nurses outlined in the Consensus Model, professional organizations have established standards and competencies for each advanced practice role:

- Accreditation Commission for Midwifery Education: *Criteria for Programmatic Accreditation* (2010)

- American Academy of Nurse Practitioners: *Standards of Practice for Nurse Practitioners* (2007)

- American Association of Nurse Anesthetists: *Scope and Standards for Nurse Anesthesia Practice* (2007)

- American College of Nurse-Midwives:

  - *Core Competencies for Basic Midwifery Practice* (2008)

  - *Standards for the Practice of Midwifery* (2009)

- Council on Accreditation of Nurse Anesthesia Educational Programs: *Competencies and Curricular Models* (2009)

- National Organization of Nurse Practitioner Faculties: *Domains and Core Competencies of Nurse Practitioner Practice* (2006)

- National Association of Clinical Nurse Specialists:

  - *Organizing Framework and CNS Core Competencies* (2008)

  - *Core Practice Doctorate Clinical Nurse Specialist (CNS) Competencies* (2009)

Nurses in Advocacy and Society

Advocacy is a fundamental aspect of nursing practice. Registered nurses have long served as healthcare consumer advocates and used grassroots networking to influence social and political leaders and other advocates. Registered nurses firmly believe it is their obligation to help improve societal conditions related to healthcare consumer care, health, and wellness. Such issues have included protective labor laws, minimum wage, communicable disease programs, immunizations, well-baby and child care, women's health, curbing violence, reproductive health, end-of-life care, universal health care, social security, Medicare and Medicaid, the financing and reimbursement of health care, healthcare reform, ethics, mental health parity, confidentiality, workplace safety, and healthcare consumer rights.

There is ample need for professional nurses to continue advocacy and lobbying. These efforts include the evaluation and restructuring of health care, reimbursement and value of nursing care, funding for nursing education, the role of nursing in health and medical homes, comparative effectiveness, and advances in health information technology. Nurses will continue to remain strong advocates for healthcare consumers, their care, and health care.

The Progression of Nursing Education

ANA's long-held position is that the baccalaureate degree is the entry degree into nursing. But nursing's educational track to professional and career growth is not linear, and while there is an explicit progression of educational degrees, there is considerable flexibility in how the progression is achieved. Educational bodies are establishing entry-into-practice master's programs, associate's degree to baccalaureate or master's degree programs, and most notably second-degree baccalaureate programs.

Two new degrees have been introduced by the American Association of Colleges of Nursing (AACN) since 2004. The Doctor of Nursing Practice (DNP) was proposed as a generic clinical degree associated with practice-based nursing, and has been proposed by AACN to be the graduate degree for advanced nursing practice or specialty preparation by 2015 (AACN, 2004). The second degree is the Clinical Nurse Leader (CNL), described as an "advanced generalist" educated at the graduate level. A defining feature of the CNL role is an emphasis on health promotion, risk reduction, and population-based health care (AACN, 2008).

IOM Influences on the Quality and Environment of Nursing Practice

To address issues in health care, the Institute of Medicine, a branch of the National Academy of Sciences, commissions reports on specific topics. While the IOM does not necessarily represent nursing, it does involve nurses in its work. Its reports and other publications are directed to universal medical practice, and sometimes explicitly to nursing, and provide a framework for systematic positive change in healthcare services.

In 1999, the Quality of Health Care in America Committee released the first and arguably most pivotal report, *To Err is Human: Building a Safer Health System*, which suggests that harm done to healthcare consumers in a profession that strives to "First, do no harm" is unacceptable. One of the most influential and paradigm-shifting conclusions of the report was that individuals and reckless behavior played only a small part in patient safety violations, and that faulty systems in which people were set up for failure were more problematic.

A second report by the committee in 2001, *Crossing the Quality Chasm: A New Health System for the 21st Century*, urges a fundamental, sweeping redesign of the entire health system. Incremental change was not enough. The committee suggested that such a system would not only improve patient safety and quality outcomes, but would also retain more health professionals who felt their contributions were making a satisfactory impact on those under their care.

Keeping Patients Safe: Transforming the Work Environment of Nurses is a key report for nurses; it considers how their interaction with their workplace helps or hinders patient care. The report reviews evidence on the work and work environments of nurses, and takes into account the behavioral traits of nurses, the organizational practices and culture, and the structural and engineering traits of the workplace. The report identifies components of the workplace most influential on nursing and patient outcomes—leadership and management, the workforce, work processes, and organizational culture—and proposes changes to these components that would lead to better outcomes for patients and nurses (IOM, 2004).

The connection between the nurse's work environment and patient mortality and failure to rescue was demonstrated by Aiken et al. (2008). Patients in hospitals with a better practice environment (characterized by nursing foundations for quality of care, nurse manager ability, leadership, and support, and collegial nurse–physician relations) fared far better than patients in hospitals with poor practice environments. To date, few work environments have achieved all of the IOM recommendations from 2004. The healthcare industry must alter the work environment of nurses to allow them to meet their social responsibility for healthcare consumer safety.

Integrating the Science and Art of Nursing

Nursing is a learned profession built on a core body of knowledge that reflects its dual components of science and art. Nursing requires judgment and skill based on principles of the biological, physical, behavioral, and social sciences. Nursing is a scientific discipline as well as a profession. Registered nurses employ critical thinking to integrate objective data with knowledge gained from an assessment of the subjective experiences of healthcare consumers. Registered nurses use critical thinking to apply the best available evidence and research data to diagnosis and treatment. Nurses continually evaluate quality and effectiveness of nursing practice and seek to optimize outcomes.

The Science of Nursing

The science of nursing is based on an analytical framework of critical thinking known as the nursing process, comprised of assessment, diagnosis, outcomes identification, planning, implementation, and evaluation. These steps serve as the foundation of clinical decision-making and support evidence-based practice. Wherever they practice, registered nurses use the nursing process and other types of critical thinking to respond to the needs of the populations they serve, and use strategies that support optimal outcomes most appropriate to the healthcare consumer or situation, being mindful of resource utilization.

Nurses as scientists rely on evidence to guide their policies and practices, but also as a way of quantifying the nurses' impact on the health outcomes of healthcare consumers. An example of ANA leadership in this area is the National Database of Nursing Quality Indicators (NDNQI®), a repository for nursing-sensitive indicators. NDNQI is the only database containing data collected at the nursing unit level.

The Art of Nursing

The art of nursing is based on caring and respect for human dignity. A compassionate approach to patient care carries a mandate to provide that care competently. Competent care is provided and accomplished through both independent practice and partnerships. Collaboration may be with other colleagues or with the individuals seeking support or assistance with their healthcare needs. Central to the nursing practice is the art of caring, which is represented in the personal relationship that the nurse enters with the patient. The art of caring goes beyond the emotional connections of humans to the ability to respond to the human aspects of health and illness within the critical moment to promote healing and calm (Watson 1999, 2008).

The art of nursing embraces dynamic processes that affect the human person, including, for example, spirituality, healing, empathy, mutual respect, and compassion. These intangible aspects foster health. Nursing embraces healing. Healing is fostered by compassion, helping, listening, mentoring, coaching, teaching, exploring, being present, supporting, touching, intuition, empathy, service, cultural competence, tolerance, acceptance, nurturing, mutually creating, and conflict resolution.

Nursing focuses on the promotion and maintenance of health and the prevention or resolution of disease, illness, or disability. The nursing needs of human beings are identified from a holistic perspective and are met in the context of a culturally sensitive, caring, personal relationship. Nursing includes the diagnosis and treatment of human responses to actual or potential health problems. Registered nurses employ practices that are restorative, supportive, and promotive in nature.

- *Restorative* practices modify the impact of illness or disease.

- *Supportive* practices are oriented toward modification of relationships or the practice environment to support health.

- *Promotive* practices mobilize healthy patterns of living, foster personal and family development, and support self-defined goals of individuals, families, communities, and populations.

Nursing's Societal and Ethical Dimensions

Nursing is responsive to the changing needs of society and the expanding knowledge base of its theoretical and scientific domains. One of nursing's objectives is to achieve positive healthcare consumer outcomes that maximize one's quality of life across the entire lifespan. Registered nurses facilitate the interprofessional and comprehensive care provided by healthcare professionals, paraprofessionals, and volunteers. In other instances, nurses engage in consultation with other colleagues to inform decision-making and planning to meet healthcare consumer needs. Registered nurses often participate in interprofessional teams in which the overlapping skills complement each member's individual efforts.

All nursing practice, regardless of specialty, role, or setting, is fundamentally independent practice. Registered nurses are accountable for nursing judgments made and actions taken in the course of their nursing practice. Therefore, the registered nurse is responsible for assessing individual competence and is committed to the process of lifelong learning. Registered nurses develop and maintain current knowledge and skills through formal and continuing education and seek certification when it is available in their areas of practice.

Registered nurses are bound by a professional code of ethics (ANA, 2001) and regulate themselves as individuals through a collegial process of peer review of practice. Peer evaluation fosters the refinement of knowledge, skills, and clinical decision-making at all levels and in all areas of clinical practice. Self-regulation by the profession of nursing assures quality of performance, which is the heart of nursing's social contract (ANA, 2010).

Registered nurses and members of various professions exchange knowledge and ideas about how to deliver high-quality health care, resulting in overlaps and constantly changing professional practice boundaries. This interprofessional team collaboration involves recognition of the expertise of others within and outside one's profession and referral to those providers when appropriate. Such collaboration also involves some shared functions and a common focus on one overall mission. By necessity, nursing's scope of practice has flexible boundaries.

Registered nurses regularly evaluate safety, effectiveness, and cost in the planning and delivery of nursing care. Nurses recognize that resources are limited and unequally distributed, and that the potential for better access to care requires innovative approaches, such as treating healthcare consumers remotely. As members of a profession, registered nurses work toward equitable distribution and availability of healthcare services throughout the nation and the world.

Caring and Nursing Practice

The essence of nursing practice is caring. "It is a beautiful and mysterious power that one human being can have on another through the mere act of caring . . . A great truth, the act of caring is the first step in the power to heal." (Moffitt, in *Relationship-Based Care*, 2004).

Watson (1999, 2008) emphasizes the personal relationship between patient and nurse. She highlights the role of the nurse in defining the patient as a unique human being and stresses the importance of the connections between the nurse and patient, modeled in her Transpersonal Caring-Healing Framework.

Leininger (1988) considers care for people from a broad range of cultures. Her five theoretical assumptions on caring are:

- Care is essential for human growth and survival, and to face death.

- There can be no curing without caring.

- Expressions of care vary among all cultures of the world.

- Therapeutic nursing care can only occur when cultural care values, expressions, or practices are known and used explicitly.

- Nursing is a transcultural care profession and discipline.

Swanson (1993) builds on Watson's framework and describes five caring processes and specific techniques for putting them into practice. The first two processes are internal processes of providing care; the other three are action processes.

- *Maintaining Belief*: Maintaining belief in persons and their capacity to make it through events and transitions

- *Knowing*: Striving to understand an event as it has meaning in the life of the other

- *Being With*: Being emotionally present to the other

- *Doing For*: Doing for the other what they would do for themselves if it were possible

- *Enabling and Informing*: Facilitating the other's passage through life transitions and unfamiliar events

Continued Commitment to the Profession

A continued commitment to the nursing profession requires a nurse to remain involved in continuous learning and strengthening individual practice within varied practice settings. This may include civic activities, membership in and support of professional associations, collective bargaining, and workplace advocacy. The code of ethics (ANA, 2001) serves as the ethical framework in nursing regardless of practice setting or role, and provides guidance for the future.

Nurses promote the health of the individual and society regardless of cultural background, value system, religious belief, gender, sexual identity, or disability. Nurses commit to their profession by utilizing their skills, knowledge, and abilities to act as visionaries, promoting safe practice environments, and supporting resourceful, accessible, and cost-effective delivery of health care to serve the ever-changing needs of the population.

Professional Trends and Issues

Despite spending more on health care than any other nation, the United States ranks 42nd in the world in life expectancy (Trust for America's Health, 2009). A reformed healthcare system focused on primary care, prevention, and chronic disease management can alleviate the financial and social costs of treating preventable and chronic diseases. Interprofessional teams and coordination of care across the illness trajectory will be key components in the new system—arenas in which nurses are familiar and have demonstrated their value. Nurses at all levels are positioned to play key roles in a reformed and restructured care delivery system, such as:

- Coordinating healthcare consumers' transitions between healthcare delivery systems and settings (e.g., from hospital to rehabilitation to home)

- Monitoring and managing healthcare consumers with chronic disease

- Promoting wellness and providing preventive health care

- Providing individualized care in nurse-managed health centers

- Participating in the "medical home" ("healthcare home") model for care management

- Utilizing advanced practice registered nurses to the fullest extent of their scope of practice consistent with education and competencies.

The nursing shortage looms as the greatest challenge to nurses to fill their critical role in health care. The aging nursing workforce, coupled with aging baby boomers, has created an imminent crisis in which record demand is timed to occur as nurses retire (Curtin, 2007). As more students are recruited into nursing, schools struggle to increase capacity. Faculty shortages—related to aging faculty, length of time to complete graduate education, heavy workload, and low salaries—severely hamper attempts by nursing schools to expand. Concern over the worsening shortage has provided the impetus for a number of innovative efforts to increase nursing capacity, including strategic partnerships to align and leverage stakeholder resources, increasing faculty capacity through accelerated programs and joint positions, redesigning nursing education, and changing policy and regulation (Joynt & Kimball, 2008).

In the face of healthcare reform and the nursing shortage, IOM and the Robert Wood Johnson Foundation have established a major initiative with the intent of "reconceptualizing the role of nurses within the context of the entire workforce, the shortage, societal issues, and current and future technology" (RWJF & IOM, 2009). The value of registered nurses in patient safety and positive patient outcomes in hospital settings is well demonstrated (Kane, Shamilyan, Mueller, Duval, & Wilt, 2007).

As healthcare reform evolves, nurses may experience greater opportunities to function within their full scope of practice across various settings. A reformed healthcare system will provide much needed incentives and financial support for utilizing nurses in various roles and promoting a full scope of practice, and eliminate the current payment practices that create barriers to innovative and effective models of practice and care delivery.

Employers are correcting workplace problems in an attempt to retain nurses. Safe patient handling, shift and scheduling options, integration of technology supports into practice, and alternative roles in the healthcare setting have enabled nurses to remain in the workplace.

As the nurse of the future evolves, so must nursing education. Curricula must be designed to adequately prepare competent entry-level nurses. The nurse shortage and program capacity limits demand efficient educational processes. Online, virtual, simulated, and competency-based learning are attempts to expand opportunities to students and increase efficiency. However, design should be based on evidence more than tradition so that the nurse graduate is prepared to provide safe and competent care.

Nursing as a profession continues to face dilemmas in entry into practice, the autonomy of advanced practice, continued competence, multistate licensure, and the appropriate educational credentials for professional certification. Registered nurses have a professional responsibility to maintain competence in their area of practice. Employers who provide opportunities for professional development and continuing education promote a positive practice environment in which nurses can maintain and enhance skills and competencies.

Technology offers a better work environment for nurses when designed and implemented in a manner that supports nurses' work. These work environments can include conventional locations—hospitals, clinics, and healthcare consumer homes—as well as virtual spaces such as online discussion groups, email, interactive video, and virtual interaction. Ideally, technology eliminates redundancy and duplication of documentation; reduces errors; eliminates interruptions for missing supplies, equipment, and medications; and eases access to data, thereby allowing the nurse more time with the patient (Pamela Cipriano, PhD, RN, FAAN, in IOM, 2009). The incorporation of technologies, however, is not without risk, and demands diligence by registered nurses to consider the impact on the scope of nursing practice and the ethical implications for healthcare consumers as well as the nurse.

The healthcare industry has been challenged to improve patient safety, patient and practitioner satisfaction, patient outcomes, and the profitability of the healthcare organization (Kennedy, 2003). In 1999 IOM described the nation's healthcare system as fractured, prone to errors, and detrimental to safe patient care. IOM has identified six aims for improvement so that the healthcare system is: safe, effective, patient-centered, timely, efficient, and equitable (IOM, 2001).

Whatever the practice venue, in the next decade registered nurses will continue to partner with others to advance the nation's health through many initiatives, such as *Healthy People 2020*. Such partnerships truly reflect the definition of nursing and illustrate the essential features of contemporary nursing practice:

- A caring relationship that facilitates health and healing

- Attention to the range of human experiences and responses to health, disease, and illness in the physical and social environments

- Integration of objective data with knowledge gained from an appreciation of the healthcare consumer's or group's subjective experience

- Application of scientific knowledge to diagnosis and treatment through the use of judgment and critical thinking

- Advancement of professional nursing knowledge through scholarly inquiry

- Influence on social and public policy to promote social justice (ANA, 2010)

Summary of the Scope of Nursing Practice

The dynamic nature of the healthcare practice environment and the growing body of nursing research provide both the impetus and the opportunity for nursing to ensure competent nursing practice in all settings for all healthcare consumers and to promote ongoing professional development that enhances the quality of nursing practice. *Nursing: Scope and Standards of Practice, Second Edition*, assists that process by delineating the professional scope and standards of practice and responsibilities of all professional registered nurses engaged in nursing practice, regardless of setting. As such, it can serve as a basis for:

- Quality improvement systems

- Regulatory systems

- Healthcare reimbursement and financing methodologies

- Development and evaluation of nursing service delivery systems and organizational structures

- Certification activities

- Position descriptions and performance appraisals

- Agency policies, procedures, and protocols

- Educational offerings

- Establishing the legal standard of care

To best serve the public's health and the nursing profession, nursing must continue its efforts to establish the Standards of Professional Nursing Practice. Nursing also must examine how the Standards of Professional Nursing Practice can be disseminated and used most effectively to enhance and promote the quality of practice. In addition, the Standards of Professional Nursing Practice must be continually evaluated and revised as necessary.

The dynamic healthcare practice environment and the growing body of nursing research provide both the impetus and the opportunity for nursing to ensure competent nursing practice in all settings for all healthcare consumers and to promote ongoing professional development that enhances the quality of nursing practice.

Standards of Professional Nursing Practice

Significance of Standards

The Standards of Professional Nursing Practice are authoritative statements of the duties that all registered nurses, regardless of role, population, or specialty, are expected to perform competently. The standards published herein may be utilized as evidence of the standard of care, with the understanding that application of the standards is context dependent. The standards are subject to change with the dynamics of the nursing profession, as new patterns of professional practice are developed and accepted by the nursing profession and the public. In addition, specific conditions and clinical circumstances may also affect the application of the standards at a given time, e.g., during a natural disaster. The standards are subject to formal, periodic review and revision. (See page 87 for information of this review and revision process.)

The Standards of Professional Nursing Practice are authoritative statements of the duties that all registered nurses, regardless of role, population, or specialty, are expected to perform competently. The standards published herein:

- May be utilized as evidence of the standard of care, with the understanding that application of the standards is context dependent

- Are subject to change with the dynamics of the nursing profession, as new patterns of professional practice are developed and accepted by the nursing profession and the public, and

- Are subject to formal, periodic review and revision.

The competencies that accompany each standard may be evidence of compliance with the corresponding standard. The list of competencies is not exhaustive for a given standard. Whether a particular standard or competency applies depends upon the circumstances.

Standards of Practice

Standard 1. Assessment

The registered nurse collects comprehensive data pertinent to the healthcare consumer's health and/or the situation.

COMPETENCIES

The registered nurse:

- Collects comprehensive data including but not limited to physical, functional, psychosocial, emotional, cognitive, sexual, cultural, age-related, environmental, spiritual/transpersonal, and economic assessments in a systematic and ongoing process while honoring the uniqueness of the person.

- Elicits the healthcare consumer's values, preferences, expressed needs, and knowledge of the healthcare situation.

- Involves the healthcare consumer, family, and other healthcare providers as appropriate, in holistic data collection.

- Identifies barriers (e.g., psychosocial, literacy, financial, cultural) to effective communication and makes appropriate adaptations.

- Recognizes the impact of personal attitudes, values, and beliefs.

- Assesses family dynamics and impact on healthcare consumer health and wellness.

- Prioritizes data collection based on the healthcare consumer's immediate condition, or the anticipated needs of the healthcare consumer or situation.

- Uses appropriate evidence-based assessment techniques, instruments, and tools.

- Synthesizes available data, information, and knowledge relevant to the situation to identify patterns and variances.

- Applies ethical, legal, and privacy guidelines and policies to the collection, maintenance, use, and dissemination of data and information.

- Recognizes the healthcare consumer as the authority on her or his own health by honoring their care preferences.

- Documents relevant data in a retrievable format.

ADDITIONAL COMPETENCIES FOR THE GRADUATE-LEVEL PREPARED SPECIALTY NURSE AND THE APRN

The graduate-level prepared specialty nurse or the advanced practice registered nurse:

- Initiates and interprets diagnostic tests and procedures relevant to the healthcare consumer's current status.

- Assesses the effect of interactions among individuals, family, community, and social systems on health and illness.

Standard 2. Diagnosis

The registered nurse analyzes the assessment data to determine the diagnoses or the issues.

COMPETENCIES

The registered nurse:

- Derives the diagnoses or issues from assessment data.

- Validates the diagnoses or issues with the healthcare consumer, family, and other healthcare providers when possible and appropriate.

- Identifies actual or potential risks to the healthcare consumer's health and safety or barriers to health, which may include but are not limited to interpersonal, systematic, or environmental circumstances.

- Uses standardized classification systems and clinical decision support tools, when available, in identifying diagnoses.

- Documents diagnoses or issues in a manner that facilitates the determination of the expected outcomes and plan.

ADDITIONAL COMPETENCIES FOR THE GRADUATE-LEVEL PREPARED SPECIALTY NURSE AND THE APRN

The graduate-level prepared specialty nurse or the advanced practice registered nurse:

- Systematically compares and contrasts clinical findings with normal and abnormal variations and developmental events in formulating a differential diagnosis.

- Utilizes complex data and information obtained during interview, examination, and diagnostic processes in identifying diagnoses.

- Assists staff in developing and maintaining competency in the diagnostic process.

Standard 3. Outcomes Identification

The registered nurse identifies expected outcomes for a plan individualized to the healthcare consumer or the situation.

COMPETENCIES

The registered nurse:

- Involves the healthcare consumer, family, healthcare providers, and others in formulating expected outcomes when possible and appropriate.

- Derives culturally appropriate expected outcomes from the diagnoses.

- Considers associated risks, benefits, costs, current scientific evidence, expected trajectory of the condition, and clinical expertise when formulating expected outcomes.

- Defines expected outcomes in terms of the healthcare consumer, healthcare consumer culture, values, and ethical considerations.

- Includes a time estimate for the attainment of expected outcomes.

- Develops expected outcomes that facilitate continuity of care.

- Modifies expected outcomes according to changes in the status of the healthcare consumer or evaluation of the situation.

- Documents expected outcomes as measurable goals.

ADDITIONAL COMPETENCIES FOR THE GRADUATE-LEVEL PREPARED SPECIALTY NURSE AND THE APRN

The graduate-level prepared specialty nurse or the advanced practice registered nurse:

- Identifies expected outcomes that incorporate scientific evidence and are achievable through implementation of evidence-based practices.

- Identifies expected outcomes that incorporate cost and clinical effectiveness, healthcare consumer satisfaction, and continuity and consistency among providers.

- Differentiates outcomes that require care process interventions from those that require system-level interventions.

Standard 4. Planning

The registered nurse develops a plan that prescribes strategies and alternatives to attain expected outcomes.

COMPETENCIES

The registered nurse:

- Develops an individualized plan in partnership with the person, family, and others considering the person's characteristics or situation, including, but not limited to, values, beliefs, spiritual and health practices, preferences, choices, developmental level, coping style, culture and environment, and available technology.

- Establishes the plan priorities with the healthcare consumer, family, and others as appropriate.

- Includes strategies in the plan that address each of the identified diagnoses or issues. These may include, but are not limited to, strategies for:

  - Promotion and restoration of health;

  - Prevention of illness, injury, and disease;

  - The alleviation of suffering; and

  - Supportive care for those who are dying.

- Includes strategies for health and wholeness across the lifespan.

- Provides for continuity in the plan.

- Incorporates an implementation pathway or timeline in the plan.

- Considers the economic impact of the plan on the healthcare consumer, family, caregivers, or other affected parties.

- Integrates current scientific evidence, trends and research.

- Utilizes the plan to provide direction to other members of the healthcare team.

- Explores practice settings and safe space and time for the nurse and the healthcare consumer to explore suggested, potential, and alternative options.

- Defines the plan to reflect current statutes, rules and regulations, and standards.

- Modifies the plan according to the ongoing assessment of the healthcare consumer's response and other outcome indicators.

- Documents the plan in a manner that uses standardized language or recognized terminology.

ADDITIONAL COMPETENCIES FOR THE GRADUATE-LEVEL PREPARED SPECIALTY NURSE AND THE APRN

The graduate-level prepared specialty nurse or the advanced practice registered nurse:

- Identifies assessment strategies, diagnostic strategies, and therapeutic interventions that reflect current evidence, including data, research, literature, and expert clinical knowledge.

- Selects or designs strategies to meet the multifaceted needs of complex healthcare consumers.

- Includes the synthesis of healthcare consumers' values and beliefs regarding nursing and medical therapies in the plan.

- Leads the design and development of interprofessional processes to address the identified diagnosis or issue.

- Actively participates in the development and continuous improvement of systems that support the planning process.

Standard 5. Implementation

The registered nurse implements the identified plan.

COMPETENCIES

The registered nurse:

- Partners with the person, family, significant others, and caregivers as appropriate to implement the plan in a safe, realistic, and timely manner.

- Demonstrates caring behaviors toward healthcare consumers, significant others, and groups of people receiving care.

- Utilizes technology to measure, record, and retrieve healthcare consumer data, implement the nursing process, and enhance nursing practice

- Utilizes evidence-based interventions and treatments specific to the diagnosis or problem.

- Provides holistic care that addresses the needs of diverse populations across the lifespan.

- Advocates for health care that is sensitive to the needs of healthcare consumers, with particular emphasis on the needs of diverse populations.

- Applies appropriate knowledge of major health problems and cultural diversity in implementing the plan of care.

- Applies available healthcare technologies to maximize access and optimize outcomes for healthcare consumers.

- Utilizes community resources and systems to implement the plan.

- Collaborates with healthcare providers from diverse backgrounds to implement and integrate the plan.

- Accommodates for different styles of communication used by healthcare consumers, families, and healthcare providers.

- Integrates traditional and complementary healthcare practices as appropriate.

- Implements the plan in a timely manner in accordance with patient safety goals.

- Promotes the healthcare consumer's capacity for the optimal level of participation and problem-solving.

- Documents implementation and any modifications, including changes or omissions, of the identified plan

ADDITIONAL COMPETENCIES FOR THE GRADUATE-LEVEL PREPARED SPECIALTY NURSE AND THE APRN

The graduate-level prepared specialty nurse or the advanced practice registered nurse:

- Facilitates utilization of systems, organizations, and community resources to implement the plan.

- Supports collaboration with nursing and other colleagues to implement the plan.

- Incorporates new knowledge and strategies to initiate change in nursing care practices if desired outcomes are not achieved.

- Assumes responsibility for the safe and efficient implementation of the plan.

- Use advanced communication skills to promote relationships between nurses and healthcare consumers, to provide a context for open discussion of the healthcare consumer's experiences, and to improve healthcare consumer outcomes.

- Actively participates in the development and continuous improvement of systems that support the implementation of the plan.

Standard 5A. Coordination of Care

The registered nurse coordinates care delivery.

COMPETENCIES

The registered nurse:

- Organizes the components of the plan.

- Manages a healthcare consumer's care in order to maximize independence and quality of life.

- Assists the healthcare consumer in identifying options for alternative care.

- Communicates with the healthcare consumer, family, and system during transitions in care.

- Advocates for the delivery of dignified and humane care by the interprofessional team.

- Documents the coordination of care.

ADDITIONAL COMPETENCIES FOR THE GRADUATE-LEVEL PREPARED SPECIALTY NURSE AND THE APRN

The graduate-level prepared specialty nurse or the advanced practice registered nurse:

- Provides leadership in the coordination of interprofessional health care for integrated delivery of healthcare consumer care services.

- Synthesizes data and information to prescribe necessary system and community support measures, including modifications of surroundings.

Standard 5B. Health Teaching and Health Promotion

The registered nurse employs strategies to promote health and a safe environment.

COMPETENCIES

The registered nurse:

- Provides health teaching that addresses such topics as healthy life-styles, risk-reducing behaviors, developmental needs, activities of daily living, and preventive self-care.

- Uses health promotion and health teaching methods appropriate to the situation and the healthcare consumer's values, beliefs, health practices, developmental level, learning needs, readiness and ability to learn, language preference, spirituality, culture, and socioeconomic status.

- Seeks opportunities for feedback and evaluation of the effectiveness of the strategies used.

- Uses information technologies to communicate health promotion and disease prevention information to the healthcare consumer in a variety of settings.

- Provides healthcare consumers with information about intended effects and potential adverse effects of proposed therapies.

ADDITIONAL COMPETENCIES FOR THE GRADUATE-LEVEL PREPARED SPECIALTY NURSE AND THE APRN

The graduate-level prepared specialty nurse or the advanced practice registered nurse:

- Synthesizes empirical evidence on risk behaviors, learning theories, behavioral change theories, motivational theories, epidemiology, and other related theories and frameworks when designing health education information and programs.

- Conducts personalized health teaching and counseling considering comparative effectiveness research recommendations.

Continued ▶

- Designs health information and healthcare consumer education appropriate to the healthcare consumer's developmental level, learning needs, readiness to learn, and cultural values and beliefs.

- Evaluates health information resources, such as the Internet, in the area of practice for accuracy, readability, and comprehensibility to help healthcare consumers access quality health information.

- Engages consumer alliances and advocacy groups, as appropriate, in health teaching and health promotion activities.

- Provides anticipatory guidance to individuals, families, groups, and communities to promote health and prevent or reduce the risk of health problems.

Standard 5C. Consultation

The graduate-level prepared specialty nurse or advanced practice registered nurse provides consultation to influence the identified plan, enhance the abilities of others, and effect change.

COMPETENCIES FOR THE GRADUATE-LEVEL PREPARED SPECIALTY NURSE AND THE APRN

The graduate-level prepared specialty nurse or the advanced practice registered nurse:

- Synthesizes clinical data, theoretical frameworks, and evidence when providing consultation.

- Facilitates the effectiveness of a consultation by involving the health-care consumers and stakeholders in decision-making and negotiating role responsibilities.

- Communicates consultation recommendations.

Standard 5D. Prescriptive Authority and Treatment

The advanced practice registered nurse uses prescriptive authority, procedures, referrals, treatments, and therapies in accordance with state and federal laws and regulations.

COMPETENCIES FOR THE ADVANCED PRACTICE REGISTERED NURSE

The advanced practice registered nurse:

- Prescribes evidence-based treatments, therapies, and procedures considering the healthcare consumer's comprehensive healthcare needs.

- Prescribes pharmacologic agents based on a current knowledge of pharmacology and physiology.

- Prescribes specific pharmacological agents or treatments according to clinical indicators, the healthcare consumer's status and needs, and the results of diagnostic and laboratory tests.

- Evaluates therapeutic and potential adverse effects of pharmacological and nonpharmacological treatments.

- Provides healthcare consumers with information about intended effects and potential adverse effects of proposed prescriptive therapies.

- Provides information about costs and alternative treatments and procedures, as appropriate.

- Evaluates and incorporates complementary and alternative therapy into education and practice.

Standard 6. Evaluation

The registered nurse evaluates progress toward attainment of outcomes.

COMPETENCIES

The registered nurse:

- Conducts a systematic, ongoing, and criterion-based evaluation of the outcomes in relation to the structures and processes prescribed by the plan of care and the indicated timeline.

- Collaborates with the healthcare consumer and others involved in the care or situation in the evaluation process.

- Evaluates, in partnership with the healthcare consumer, the effectiveness of the planned strategies in relation to the healthcare consumer's responses and the attainment of the expected outcomes.

- Uses ongoing assessment data to revise the diagnoses, outcomes, the plan, and the implementation as needed.

- Disseminates the results to the healthcare consumer, family, and others involved, in accordance with federal and state regulations.

- Participates in assessing and assuring the responsible and appropriate use of interventions in order to minimize unwarranted or unwanted treatment and healthcare consumer suffering.

- Documents the results of the evaluation.

ADDITIONAL COMPETENCIES FOR THE GRADUATE-LEVEL PREPARED SPECIALTY NURSE AND THE APRN

The graduate-level prepared specialty nurse or the advanced practice registered nurse:

- Evaluates the accuracy of the diagnosis and the effectiveness of the interventions and other variables in relation to the healthcare consumer's attainment of expected outcomes.

Continued ▶

- Synthesizes the results of the evaluation to determine the effect of the plan on healthcare consumers, families, groups, communities, and institutions.

- Adapts the plan of care for the trajectory of treatment according to evaluation of response.

- Uses the results of the evaluation to make or recommend process or structural changes including policy, procedure, or protocol revision, as appropriate.

Standards of Professional Performance

Standard 7. Ethics

The registered nurse practices ethically.

COMPETENCIES

The registered nurse:

- Uses *Code of Ethics for Nurses with Interpretive Statements* (ANA, 2001) to guide practice.

- Delivers care in a manner that preserves and protects healthcare consumer autonomy, dignity, rights, values, and beliefs.

- Recognizes the centrality of the healthcare consumer and family as core members of any healthcare team.

- Upholds healthcare consumer confidentiality within legal and regulatory parameters.

- Assists healthcare consumers in self determination and informed decision-making.

- Maintains a therapeutic and professional healthcare consumer–nurse relationship within appropriate professional role boundaries.

- Contributes to resolving ethical issues involving healthcare consumers, colleagues, community groups, systems, and other stakeholders.

- Takes appropriate action regarding instances of illegal, unethical, or inappropriate behavior that can endanger or jeopardize the best interests of the healthcare consumer or situation.

- Speaks up when appropriate to question healthcare practice when necessary for safety and quality improvement.

- Advocates for equitable healthcare consumer care.

Continued ▶

ADDITIONAL COMPETENCIES FOR THE GRADUATE-LEVEL PREPARED SPECIALTY NURSE AND THE APRN

The graduate-level prepared specialty nurse or the advanced practice registered nurse:

- Participates in interprofessional teams that address ethical risks, benefits, and outcomes.

- Provides information on the risks, benefits, and outcomes of healthcare regimens to allow informed decision-making by the healthcare consumer, including informed consent and informed refusal.

Standard 8. Education

The registered nurse attains knowledge and competence that reflects current nursing practice.

COMPETENCIES

The registered nurse:

- Participates in ongoing educational activities related to appropriate knowledge bases and professional issues.

- Demonstrates a commitment to lifelong learning through self-reflection and inquiry to address learning and personal growth needs.

- Seeks experiences that reflect current practice to maintain knowledge, skills, abilities, and judgment in clinical practice or role performance.

- Acquires knowledge and skills appropriate to the role, population, specialty, setting, role, or situation.

- Seeks formal and independent learning experiences to develop and maintain clinical and professional skills and knowledge.

- Identifies learning needs based on nursing knowledge, the various roles the nurse may assume, and the changing needs of the population.

- Participates in formal or informal consultations to address issues in nursing practice as an application of education and a knowledge base.

- Shares educational findings, experiences, and ideas with peers.

- Contributes to a work environment conducive to the education of healthcare professionals.

- Maintains professional records that provide evidence of competence and lifelong learning.

Continued ▶

ADDITIONAL COMPETENCIES FOR THE GRADUATE-LEVEL PREPARED SPECIALTY NURSE AND THE APRN

The graduate-level prepared specialty nurse or the advanced practice registered nurse:

- Uses current healthcare research findings and other evidence to expand clinical knowledge, skills, abilities, and judgment, to enhance role performance, and to increase knowledge of professional issues.

Standard 9. Evidence-Based Practice and Research

The registered nurse integrates evidence and research findings into practice.

COMPETENCIES

The registered nurse:

- Utilizes current evidence-based nursing knowledge, including research findings, to guide practice.

- Incorporates evidence when initiating changes in nursing practice.

- Participates, as appropriate to education level and position, in the formulation of evidence-based practice through research.

- Shares personal or third-party research findings with colleagues and peers.

ADDITIONAL COMPETENCIES FOR THE GRADUATE-LEVEL PREPARED SPECIALTY NURSE AND THE APRN

The graduate-level prepared specialty nurse or the advanced practice registered nurse:

- Contributes to nursing knowledge by conducting or synthesizing research and other evidence that discovers, examines, and evaluates current practice, knowledge, theories, criteria, and creative approaches to improve healthcare outcomes.

- Promotes a climate of research and clinical inquiry.

- Disseminates research findings through activities such as presentations, publications, consultation, and journal clubs.

Standard 10. Quality of Practice

The registered nurse contributes to quality nursing practice.

COMPETENCIES

The registered nurse:

- Demonstrates quality by documenting the application of the nursing process in a responsible, accountable, and ethical manner.

- Uses creativity and innovation to enhance nursing care.

- Participates in quality improvement. Activities may include:

  - Identifying aspects of practice important for quality monitoring;

  - Using indicators to monitor quality, safety, and effectiveness of nursing practice;

  - Collecting data to monitor quality and effectiveness of nursing practice;

  - Analyzing quality data to identify opportunities for improving nursing practice;

  - Formulating recommendations to improve nursing practice or outcomes;

  - Implementing activities to enhance the quality of nursing practice;

  - Developing, implementing, and/or evaluating policies, procedures, and guidelines to improve the quality of practice;

  - Participating on and/or leading interprofessional teams to evaluate clinical care or health services;

  - Participating in and/or leading efforts to minimize costs and unnecessary duplication;

  - Identifying problems that occur in day-to-day work routines in order to correct process inefficiencies;*

  - Analyzing factors related to quality, safety, and effectiveness,

---

*BHE/MONE, 2006.

- Analyzing organizational systems for barriers to quality healthcare consumer outcomes; and

- Implementing processes to remove or weaken barriers within organizational systems.

ADDITIONAL COMPETENCIES FOR THE GRADUATE-LEVEL PREPARED SPECIALTY NURSE AND THE APRN

The graduate-level prepared specialty nurse or the advanced practice registered nurse:

- Provides leadership in the design and implementation of quality improvements.

- Designs innovations to effect change in practice and improve health outcomes.

- Evaluates the practice environment and quality of nursing care rendered in relation to existing evidence.

- Identifies opportunities for the generation and use of research and evidence.

- Obtains and maintains professional certification if it is available in the area of expertise.

- Uses the results of quality improvement to initiate changes in nursing practice and the healthcare delivery system.

Standard 11. Communication

The registered nurse communicates effectively in a variety of formats in all areas of practice.

COMPETENCIES

The registered nurse:

- Assesses communication format preferences of healthcare consumers, families, and colleagues.*

- Assesses her or his own communication skills in encounters with healthcare consumers, families, and colleagues.*

- Seeks continuous improvement of communication and conflict resolution skills.*

- Conveys information to healthcare consumers, families, the interprofessional team, and others in communication formats that promote accuracy.

- Questions the rationale supporting care processes and decisions when they do not appear to be in the best interest of the patient.*

- Discloses observations or concerns related to hazards and errors in care or the practice environment to the appropriate level.

- Maintains communication with other providers to minimize risks associated with transfers and transition in care delivery.

- Contributes her or his own professional perspective in discussions with the interprofessional team.

---

*BHE/MONE, 2006.

Standard 12. Leadership

The registered nurse demonstrates leadership in the professional practice setting and the profession.

COMPETENCIES

The registered nurse:

- Oversees the nursing care given by others while retaining accountability for the quality of care given to the healthcare consumer.

- Abides by the vision, the associated goals, and the plan to implement and measure progress of an individual healthcare consumer or progress within the context of the healthcare organization.

- Demonstrates a commitment to continuous, lifelong learning and education for self and others.

- Mentors colleagues for the advancement of nursing practice, the profession, and quality health care.

- Treats colleagues with respect, trust, and dignity.*

- Develops communication and conflict resolution skills.

- Participates in professional organizations.

- Communicates effectively with the healthcare consumer and colleagues.

- Seeks ways to advance nursing autonomy and accountability.*

- Participates in efforts to influence healthcare policy involving healthcare consumers and the profession.*

---

*BHE/MONE, 2006.

Continued ▶

ADDITIONAL COMPETENCIES FOR THE GRADUATE-LEVEL PREPARED SPECIALTY NURSE AND THE APRN

The graduate-level prepared specialty nurse or the advanced practice registered nurse:

- Influences decision-making bodies to improve the professional practice environment and healthcare consumer outcomes.

- Provides direction to enhance the effectiveness of the interprofessional team.

- Promotes advanced practice nursing and role development by interpreting its role for healthcare consumers, families, and others.

- Models expert practice to interprofessional team members and healthcare consumers.

- Mentors colleagues in the acquisition of clinical knowledge, skills, abilities, and judgment.

Standard 13. Collaboration

The registered nurse collaborates with healthcare consumer, family, and others in the conduct of nursing practice.

COMPETENCIES

The registered nurse:

- Partners with others to effect change and produce positive outcomes through the sharing of knowledge of the healthcare consumer and/or situation.

- Communicates with the healthcare consumer, the family, and healthcare providers regarding healthcare consumer care and the nurse's role in the provision of that care.

- Promotes conflict management and engagement.

- Participates in building consensus or resolving conflict in the context of patient care.

- Applies group process and negotiation techniques with healthcare consumers and colleagues.

- Adheres to standards and applicable codes of conduct that govern behavior among peers and colleagues to create a work environment that promotes cooperation, respect, and trust.

- Cooperates in creating a documented plan focused on outcomes and decisions related to care and delivery of services that indicates communication with healthcare consumers, families, and others.

- Engages in teamwork and team-building process.

Continued ▶

ADDITIONAL COMPETENCIES FOR THE GRADUATE-LEVEL PREPARED SPECIALTY NURSE AND THE APRN

The graduate-level prepared specialty nurse or the advanced practice registered nurse:

- Partners with other disciplines to enhance healthcare consumer outcomes through interprofessional activities, such as education, consultation, management, technological development, or research opportunities.

- Invites the contribution of the healthcare consumer, family, and team members in order to achieved optimal outcomes.

- Leads in establishing, improving, and sustaining collaborative relationships to achieve safe, quality healthcare consumer care.

- Documents plan-of-care communications, rationales for plan-of-care changes, and collaborative discussions to improve healthcare consumer outcomes.

Standard 14. Professional Practice Evaluation

The registered nurse evaluates her or his own nursing practice in relation to professional practice standards and guidelines, relevant statutes, rules, and regulations.

COMPETENCIES

The registered nurse:

- Provides age-appropriate and developmentally appropriate care in a culturally and ethnically sensitive manner.

- Engages in self-evaluation of practice on a regular basis, identifying areas of strength as well as areas in which professional growth would be beneficial.

- Obtains informal feedback regarding her or his own practice from healthcare consumers, peers, professional colleagues, and others.

- Participates in peer review as appropriate.

- Takes action to achieve goals identified during the evaluation process.

- Provides the evidence for practice decisions and actions as part of the informal and formal evaluation processes.

- Interacts with peers and colleagues to enhance her or his own professional nursing practice or role performance.

- Provides peers with formal or informal constructive feedback regarding their practice or role performance.

ADDITIONAL COMPETENCIES FOR THE GRADUATE-LEVEL PREPARED SPECIALTY NURSE AND THE APRN

The graduate-level prepared specialty nurse or the advanced practice registered nurse:

- Engages in a formal process seeking feedback regarding her or his own practice from healthcare consumers, peers, professional colleagues, and others.

Standard 15. Resource Utilization

The registered nurse utilizes appropriate resources to plan and provide nursing services that are safe, effective, and financially responsible.

COMPETENCIES

The registered nurse:

- Assesses individual healthcare consumer care needs and resources available to achieve desired outcomes.

- Identifies healthcare consumer care needs, potential for harm, complexity of the task, and desired outcome when considering resource allocation.

- Delegates elements of care to appropriate healthcare workers in accordance with any applicable legal or policy parameters or principles.

- Identifies the evidence when evaluating resources.

- Advocates for resources, including technology, that enhance nursing practice.

- Modifies practice when necessary to promote positive interaction between healthcare consumers, care providers, and technology.

- Assists the healthcare consumer and family in identifying and securing appropriate services to address needs across the healthcare continuum.

- Assists the healthcare consumer and family in factoring costs, risks, and benefits in decisions about treatment and care.

ADDITIONAL COMPETENCIES FOR THE GRADUATE-LEVEL PREPARED SPECIALTY NURSE AND THE APRN

The graduate-level prepared specialty nurse or the advanced practice registered nurse:

- Utilizes organizational and community resources to formulate inter-professional plans of care.

- Formulates innovative solutions for healthcare consumer care problems that utilize resources effectively and maintain quality.

- Designs evaluation strategies that demonstrate cost-effectiveness, cost-benefit, and efficiency factors associated with nursing practice.

Standard 16. Environmental Health

The registered nurse practices in an environmentally safe and healthy manner.

COMPETENCIES

The registered nurse:

- Attains knowledge of environmental health concepts, such as implementation of environmental health strategies.

- Promotes a practice environment that reduces environmental health risks for workers and healthcare consumers.

- Assesses the practice environment for factors such as sound, odor, noise, and light that threaten health.

- Advocates for the judicious and appropriate use of products in health care.

- Communicates environmental health risks and exposure reduction strategies to healthcare consumers, families, colleagues, and communities.

- Utilizes scientific evidence to determine if a product or treatment is an environmental threat.

- Participates in strategies to promote healthy communities.

ADDITIONAL COMPETENCIES FOR THE GRADUATE-LEVEL PREPARED SPECIALTY NURSE AND THE APRN

The graduate-level prepared specialty nurse or the advanced practice registered nurse:

- Creates partnerships that promote sustainable environmental health policies and conditions.

- Analyzes the impact of social, political, and economic influences on the environment and human health exposures.

Continued ▶

- Critically evaluates the manner in which environmental health issues are presented by the popular media.

- Advocates for implementation of environmental principles for nursing practice.

- Supports nurses in advocating for and implementing environmental principles in nursing practice.

Glossary

Advanced practice registered nurses (APRN). A nurse who has completed an accredited graduate-level education program preparing her or him for the role of certified nurse practitioner, certified registered nurse anesthetist, certified nurse-midwife, or clinical nurse specialist; has passed a national certification examination that measures the APRN role and population-focused competencies; maintains continued competence as evidenced by recertification; and is licensed to practice as an APRN. (Adapted from APRN JDG, 2008.)

Assessment. A systematic, dynamic process by which the registered nurse, through interaction with the patient, family, groups, communities, populations, and healthcare providers, collects and analyzes data. Assessment may include the following dimensions: physical, psychological, sociocultural, spiritual, cognitive, functional abilities, developmental, economic, and lifestyle.

Autonomy. The capacity of a nurse to determine her or his own actions through independent choice, including demonstration of competence, within the full scope of nursing practice.

Caregiver. A person who provides direct care for another, such as a child, dependent adult, the disabled, or the chronically ill.

Code of ethics (nursing). A list of provisions that makes explicit the primary goals, values, and obligations of the nursing profession and expresses its values, duties, and commitments to the society of which it is a part. In the United States, nurses abide by and adhere to the Code of Ethics for Nurses (ANA, 2001).

Collaboration. A professional healthcare partnership grounded in a reciprocal and respectful recognition and acceptance of: each partner's unique expertise, power, and sphere of influence and responsibilities; the commonality of goals; the mutual safeguarding of the legitimate interest of each party; and the advantages of such a relationship.

Competency. An expected and measureable level of nursing performance that integrates knowledge, skills, abilities, and judgment, based on established scientific knowledge and expectations for nursing practice.

Continuity of care. An interprofessional process that includes healthcare consumers, families, and other stakeholders in the development of a coordinated plan of care. This process facilitates the patient's transition between settings and healthcare providers, based on changing needs and available resources.

Delegation. The transfer of responsibility for the performance of a task from one individual to another while retaining accountability for the outcome. Example: the RN, in delegating a task to an assistive individual, transfers the responsibility for the performance of the task but retains professional accountability for the overall care.

Diagnosis. A clinical judgment about the healthcare consumer's response to actual or potential health conditions or needs. The diagnosis provides the basis for determination of a plan to achieve expected outcomes. Registered nurses utilize nursing and medical diagnoses depending upon educational and clinical preparation and legal authority.

Environment. The surrounding context, milieu, conditions, or atmosphere in which a registered nurse practices.

Environmental health. Aspects of human health, including quality of life, that are determined by physical, chemical, biological, social, and psychological problems in the environment. It also refers to the theory and practice of assessing, correcting, controlling, and preventing those factors in the environment that can potentially affect adversely the health of present and future generations.

Evaluation. The process of determining the progress toward attainment of expected outcomes, including the effectiveness of care.

Expected outcomes. End results that are measurable, desirable, and observable, and translate into observable behaviors.

Evidence-based practice. A scholarly and systematic problem-solving paradigm that results in the delivery of high-quality health care.

Family. Family of origin or significant others as identified by the healthcare consumer.

Graduate-level prepared specialty nurse. A registered nurse prepared at the master's or doctoral educational level who has advanced knowledge, skills, abilities, and judgment associated with one or more nursing specialties and is functioning in an advanced level as designated by elements of her or his position.

Health. An experience that is often expressed in terms of wellness and illness, and may occur in the presence or absence of disease or injury.

Healthcare consumer. The person, client, family, group, community, or population who is the focus of attention and to whom the registered nurse is providing services as sanctioned by the state regulatory bodies.

Healthcare providers. Individuals with special expertise who provide healthcare services or assistance to patients. They may include nurses, physicians, psychologists, social workers, nutritionist/dietitians, and various therapists.

Illness. The subjective experience of discomfort.

Implementation. Activities such as teaching, monitoring, providing, counseling, delegating, and coordinating.

Information. Data that are interpreted, organized, or structured.

Interprofessional. Reliant on the overlapping knowledge, skills, and abilities of each professional team member. This can drive synergistic effects by which outcomes are enhanced and become more comprehensive than a simple aggregation of the individual efforts of the team members.

Medical home. Care that uses primary care providers to ensure the delivery of coordinated, comprehensive care.

Nursing. The protection, promotion, and optimization of health and abilities, prevention of illness and injury, alleviation of suffering through the diagnosis and treatment of human response, and advocacy in the care of individuals, families, communities, and populations.

Nursing practice. The collective professional activities of nurses characterized by the interrelations of human responses, theory application, nursing actions, and outcomes.

Nursing process. A critical thinking model used by nurses that comprises the integration of the singular, concurrent actions of these six components: assessment, diagnosis, identification of outcomes, planning, implementation, and evaluation.

Patient. *See* Healthcare consumer.

Peer review. A collegial, systematic, and periodic process by which registered nurses are held accountable for practice and that fosters the refinement of one's knowledge, skills, and decision-making at all levels and in all areas of practice.

Plan. A comprehensive outline of the components that need to be addressed to attain expected outcomes.

Quality. The degree to which health services for patients, families, groups, communities, or populations increase the likelihood of desired outcomes and are consistent with current professional knowledge.

Registered nurse (RN). An individual registered or licensed by a state, commonwealth, territory, government, or other regulatory body to practice as a registered nurse.

Scope of Nursing Practice. The description of the *who, what, where, when, why*, and *how* of nursing practice that addresses the range of nursing practice activities common to all registered nurses. When considered in conjunction with the Standards of Professional Nursing Practice and the Code of Ethics for Nurses, comprehensively describes the competent level of nursing common to all registered nurses.

Standards. Authoritative statements defined and promoted by the profession by which the quality of practice, service, or education can be evaluated.

Standards of Practice. Describe a competent level of nursing care as demonstrated by the nursing process. *See also* Nursing process.

Standards of Professional Nursing Practice. Authoritative statements of the duties that all registered nurses, regardless of role, population, or specialty, are expected to perform competently.

Standards of Professional Performance. Describe a competent level of behavior in the professional role.

References and Bibliography

All URLs were retrieved on August 18, 2010.

Accreditation Commission for Midwifery Education (ACME). (2010). *Criteria for programmatic accreditation.* Silver Spring: Author. http://www.midwife.org/acmedocs/ACME.Programmatic.Criteria .Final.June.2010.pdf

American Academy of Nurse Practitioners (AANP). (2007). *Standards of practice for nurse practitioners.* Washington, DC: Author. http:// www.aanp.org/NR/rdonlyres/FE00E81B-FA96-4779-972B- 6162F04C309F/0/Standards_of_Practice112907.pdf

American Association of Colleges of Nursing (AACN). (2004). *AACN position statement on the practice doctorate in nursing.* October 2004 Washington, DC: Author.

American Association of Colleges of Nursing (AACN). (2008). *The essentials of baccalaureate education for professional nursing practice.* Washington, DC: Author.

American Association of Critical-Care Nurses (AACN). (2005). *AACN standards for establishing and maintaining healthy work environments.* Mission Viejo, CA: Author.

American Association of Nurse Anesthetists (AANA). Council on Accreditation of Nurse Anesthesia Educational Programs (COA). (n.d). *Competencies and curricular models.* Park Ridge, IL: Author. http://www.aana.com/uploadedFiles/Professional_Development/ Nurse_Anesthesia_Education/Educational_Resources/DTF_Report/ competencies.pdf

American Association of Nurse Anesthetists (AANA). (2007). *Scope and standards for nurse anesthesia practice.* Park Ridge, IL: Author. http://www.aana.com/uploadedFiles/Resources/Practice_Documents/ scope_stds_nap07_2007.pdf

American College of Nurse-Midwives (ACNM). (2008). *Core competencies for basic midwifery practice.* Silver Spring: Author. http://www.midwife. org/siteFiles/descriptive/Core_Competencies_6_07_000.pdf

American College of Nurse-Midwives (ACNM). (2009). *Standards for the practice of midwifery.* Silver Spring: Author. http://www.midwife.org/ siteFiles/descriptive/Standards_for_Practice_of_Midwifery_12_09_001 .pdf

American Journal of Nursing. (1911). Editorial comments. Room at the top. *12*(2), 85–90. (Available to subscribers only at http://journals.lww.com/ ajnonline/toc/1911/11000)

American Nurses Asssociation (ANA). (2001). *Code of Ethics for Nurses with interpretive statements.* Washington, DC: Nursesbooks.org.

American Nurses Association (ANA). (2007). *ANA principles of environmental health for nursing practice with implementation strategies.* Silver Spring, MD: Nursesbooks.org.

American Nurses Association. (2008). *Professional role competence (Position Statement).* Silver Spring, MD: Author.

American Nurses Association (ANA). (2010). *Nursing's social policy statement: The essence of the profession.* Silver Spring, MD: Nursesbooks.org.

American Nurses Credentialing Center (ANCC). (2008). *A new model for ANCC's Magnet Recognition Program.* Silver Spring, MD: Author.

APRN Joint Dialogue Group. (2008). *The Consensus Model for Advanced Practice Registered Nurses (APRN): Licensure, accreditation, certification and education.* http://www.nursingworld.org/ConsensusModelforAPRN

Benner, P. (1982). From novice to expert. *American Journal of Nursing, 82*(3), 402–407.

Board of Higher Education & Massachusetts Organization of Nurse Executives (BHE/MONE). (2006). *Creativity and connections: Building the framework for the future of nursing education. Report from the Invitational Working Session, March 23-24, 2006*. Burlington, MA: MONE. http://www.mass .edu/currentinit/documents/NursingCreativityAndConnections.pdf

Curtin, L. (2007). The perfect storm: Managed care, aging adults, and a nursing shortage. *Nursing Administration Quarterly, 31*(2), 105–114.

Gallagher-Lepak, S., & Kubsch, S. (2009). Transpersonal caring: A nursing practice guideline. *Holistic Nursing Practice, 23*, 171–182.

Hagerty, B. M. K., Lynch-Sauer, K., Patusky, K. L., & Bouwseman, M. (1993). An emerging theory of human relatedness. *Image, 25*, 291–296.

Institute of Medicine (IOM). (1999). *To err is human: Building a safer health system*. Washington, DC: National Academies Press.

Institute of Medicine (IOM). (2001). *Crossing the quality chasm*. Washington, DC: National Academies Press.

Institute of Medicine (IOM). (2003). *Health professions education: A bridge to quality*. Washington, DC: National Academies Press.

Institute of Medicine (IOM). (2004). *Keeping patients safe: Transforming the work environment of nurses*. Washington, DC: National Academies Press.

Institute of Medicine. (2009). *Forum on the Future of Nursing: Acute care.* "Technology-Enabled Nursing" and "Reactions and Questions" in Chapter 4, Technology, pgs.28–33. Washington, DC: National Academies Press. http://www.nap.edu/catalog.php?record_id=12855

Joynt J. & Kimball, B. (2008). *Blowing open the bottleneck: Designing new approaches to increase nurse education capacity*. Princeton, NJ: Robert Wood Johnson Foundation.

Kane, R.L., Shamilyan, T., Mueller, C., Duval, S. & Wilt, T.J. (2007). *Nurse staffing and quality of patient care*. Rockville, MD: Agency for Health-care Research and Quality.

Leininger, M. (1988). Leininger's Theory of Nursing: Cultural care diversity and universality. *Nursing Science Quarterly, 1*(4), 152–160.

National Association of Clinical Nurse Specialists (NACNS). (2008). *Organizing framework and CNS core competencies.* Philadelphia: Author. http://nacns .org/LinkClick.aspx?fileticket=22R8AaNmrUI%3d&tabid=139

National Association of Clinical Nurse Specialists (NACNS). (2009). *Core practice doctorate clinical nurse specialist (CNS) competencies.* Philadelphia: Author. http://www.nacns.org/LinkClick.aspx?fileticket= PAlL7o%2FjOFY%3D&tabid=36

National Organization of Nurse Practitioner Faculties. (2006). *Domains and core competencies of nurse practitioner practice.* Author. http://www .nonpf.com/associations/10789/files/DomainsandCoreComps2006.pdf

Nightingale, F. (1859). *Notes on nursing.* New York: Dover Publications.

Robert Wood Johnson Foundation (RWJF) & Institute of Medicine (IOM). (2009). *Robert Wood Johnson Foundation, Institute of Medicine launch unprecedented initiative on the future of nursing in America.* Princeton, NJ: RWJF. http://www.rwjf.org/pr/product.jsp?id=45714

Stewart, I. M. (1948). *The education of nurses: Historical foundations and modern trends.* New York: Macmillan Company.

Swanson, K. (1993). Empirical development of a middle-range theory of caring. *Nursing Research, 40*(3), 161–166.

Trust for America's Health. (2009). *Making the case: Prevention and health reform.* Washington, DC: Author. http://healthyamericans.org/assets/ files/5.20.09PreventionandReformTPs.pdf

U.S. Department of Health and Human Services (DHHS), Health Resources and Services Administration (2010). The Registered Nurse population: Initial findings from the 2008 National Sample Survey of Registered Nurses. Washington, DC: Author. http://www.bhpr.hrsa.gov/ healthworkforce/msurvey/

U.S. Department of Labor. Bureau of Labor Statistics (2010). *Occupational outlook handbook, 2010–11 edition. Registered nurses.* Washington, DC: Author. http://www.bls.gov/oco/ocos083.htm

Watson, J. (1999). *Postmodern nursing and beyond.* Edinburgh: Churchill Livingstone.

Watson, J. (2008). *Nursing: The philosophy and science of caring.* Boulder, CO: University Press of Colorado.

Appendix A.

ANA's Principles of Environmental Health for Nursing Practice (2007)

1. Knowledge of environmental health concepts is essential to nursing practice.

2. The Precautionary Principle guides nurses in their practice to use products and practices that do not harm human health or the environment and to take preventive action in the face of uncertainty.

3. Nurses have a right to work in an environment that is safe and healthy.

4. Healthy environments are sustained through multidisciplinary collaboration.

5. Choices of materials, products, technology, and practices in the environment that impact nursing practice are based on the best evidence available.

6. Approaches to promoting a healthy environment respect the diverse values, beliefs, cultures, and circumstances of patients and their families.

7. Nurses participate in assessing the quality of the environment in which they practice and live.

Continued ▶

8. Nurses, other healthcare workers, patients, and communities have the right to know relevant and timely information about the potentially harmful products, chemicals, pollutants, and hazards to which they are exposed.

9. Nurses participate in research of best practices that promote a safe and healthy environment.

10. Nurses must be supported in advocating for and implementing environmental health principles in nursing practice.

Source: ANA, 2007; p. 17.

Appendix B.

Professional Role Competence: ANA Position Statement (2008)

Summary of the ANA position on professional role competence

The public has a right to expect registered nurses to demonstrate professional competence throughout their careers. ANA believes the registered nurse is individually responsible and accountable for maintaining professional competence. The ANA further believes that it is the nursing profession's responsibility to shape and guide any process for assuring nurse competence. Regulatory agencies define minimal standards for regulation of practice to protect the public. The employer is responsible and accountable to provide an environment conducive to competent practice. Assurance of competence is the shared responsibility of the profession, individual nurses, professional organizations, credentialing and certification entities, regulatory agencies, employers, and other key stakeholders. (Issued May 29, 2008.) http://www.nursingworld .org/NursingPractice

Position Statement

Professional Role Competence

Effective Date: May 28, 2008
Status: New Position Statement
Originated By: Congress on Nursing Practice and Economics
Adopted By: ANA Board of Directors

Purpose: The purpose of this position statement is to define competence and competency in the professional role of the registered nurse within the context of today's healthcare environment. This position statement also identifies principles for addressing competence in the nursing profession. Initiatives such as the development of the scope and standards of nursing practice, creation of educational curricula, formulation of a research agenda, and revision of the model nurse practice act and other regulatory requirements demand that American Nurses Association (ANA) take a position on this important nursing issue. The work of other professional groups on this topic, i.e. National Council of State Boards of Nursing (NCSBN), nursing specialty groups, and other professional groups, has been reviewed.

Statement of ANA Position: The public has a right to expect registered nurses to demonstrate professional competence throughout their careers. ANA believes the registered nurse is individually responsible and accountable for maintaining professional competence. The ANA further believes that it is the nursing profession's responsibility to shape and guide any process for assuring nurse competence. Regulatory agencies define minimal standards for regulation of practice to protect the public. The employer is responsible and accountable to provide an environment conducive to competent practice. Assurance of competence is the shared responsibility of the profession, individual nurses, professional organizations, credentialing and certification entities, regulatory agencies, employers, and other key stakeholders.

ANA believes that in the practice of nursing, competence is definable, measurable and can be evaluated. No single evaluation method or tool can guarantee competence. Competence is situational, dynamic, and is both an outcome and an ongoing process (Competency and Credentialing Institute [CCI], 2007). Context determines what competencies are necessary. The measurement criteria included with each ANA standard of nursing practice "are key indicators of competent practice for each standard" (ANA, 2004, p. 5).

These measurement criteria need further refinement to evolve into the requisite competency statements accompanying each standard of nursing practice and professional performance.

History/previous position statements

In May 1999, the ANA Board of Directors appointed an Expert Nursing Panel on Continuing Competence with representation from the State Nurses' Associations (SNA), the ANA board, the American Nurses Foundation (ANF), and the American Academy of Nursing (AAN), the American Nurses Credentialing Center (ANCC), the Nursing Organizations Liaison Forum (NOLF), and the National Council of State Boards of Nursing (NCSBN). This group was charged to develop policy recommendations and an action plan with a proposed research agenda. In August 1999, the ANF board funded a grant titled "The Profession's Action for Continued Competence" to support this work. The ANA Board received the report of the expert panel and authorized review and comments to be sought from the Constituent Member Associations (CMA), the United American Nurses (UAN), the Congress on Nursing Practice and Economics (CNPE), and other related entities (ANA, 2000).

In 2002 the expert panel proposed the Continuing Professional Nursing Competence (CNPC) Process to the ANA House of Delegates. This proposed process incorporated the development of portfolios by individual nurses to document ongoing activities related to the demonstration of continuing competence. The resultant discussion indicated the need for further exploration of this topic.

In 2005 the ANA's Committee on Nursing Practice Standards and Guidelines began a working paper about competence and its relationship to the ANA's *Nursing: Scope and Standards of Practice* (ANA, 2004) document. This paper was presented to the Congress on Nursing Practice and Economics (CNPE) in November 2006 for continued development.

Supportive material: The ANA's *Nursing's Social Policy Statement* (2003) and *Nursing: Scope and Standards of Practice* (2004) define: "Nursing is the protection, promotion, and optimization of health and abilities, prevention of illness and injury, alleviation of suffering through the diagnosis and treatment of human response, and advocacy in the care of individuals, families, communities, and populations" (ANA, 2004, p.7). Therefore, the primary purpose for ensuring competence is the protection of the public (ANA, 2003). A secondary purpose for ensuring competence is the advancement of the profession through the continued professional development of nurses. A third purpose is to ensure the integrity of professional nursing.

The ANA's *Code of Ethics for Nurses with Interpretive Statements* (2001) states: "Individual nurses are accountable for assessing their own competence" (p. 17) and "maintenance of competence and ongoing professional growth involves the control of one's own conduct in a way that is primarily self-regarding. Competence affects one's self-respect, self-esteem, professional status and the meaningfulness of work. In all nursing roles, evaluation of one's own performance, coupled with peer review, is a means by which nursing practice can be held to the highest standards" (p.18). "The nurse owes the same duties to self and to others . . . to maintain competence, and to continue personal and professional growth" (p. 18).

Definitions and Concepts in Competence

- An individual who demonstrates *"competence"* is performing successfully at an expected level.

- A *"competency"* is an expected level of performance that integrates knowledge, skills, abilities, and judgment.

- The integration of knowledge, skills, abilities, and judgment occurs in formal, informal, and reflective learning experiences.

- Knowledge encompasses thinking; understanding of science and humanities; professional standards of practice, and insights gained from practical experiences, personal capabilities, and leadership performance.

- Skills include psychomotor, communication, interpersonal, and diagnostic skills.

- Ability is the capacity to act effectively. It requires listening, integrity, knowledge of one's strengths and weaknesses, positive self-regard, emotional intelligence, and openness to feedback.

- Judgment includes critical thinking, problem solving, ethical reasoning, and decision-making.

- Formal learning most often occurs in structured, academic, and professional development environments, while informal learning can be described as experiential insights gained in work, community, home, and other settings. Reflective learning represents the recurrent thoughtful personal self-assessment, analysis, and synthesis of strengths and opportunities for improvement. Such insights should lead to the creation of a specific plan for professional development and may become part of one's professional portfolio.

COMPETENCE AND COMPETENCY IN NURSING PRACTICE

Competent registered nurses can be influenced by the nature of the situation, which includes consideration of the setting, resources, and the person. Situations can either enhance or detract from the nurse's ability to perform. The registered nurse influences factors that facilitate and enhance competent practice. Similarly the nurse seeks to deal with barriers that constrain competent practice.

The ability to perform at the expected level requires a process of lifelong learning. Registered nurses must continually reassess their competencies and identify needs for additional knowledge, skills, personal growth, and integrative learning experiences.

The expected level of performance reflects variability depending upon context and the selected competence framework or model. Examples of such frameworks for registered nurses include, but are not limited to:

- *Nursing: Scope and Standards of Practice* (ANA, 2004)

- Specialty nursing scope and standards of practice

- Academic and professional development models (AACN, 1998)

- Benner's Novice to Expert Model (1982)

- Credentialing and privileging requirements

- Statutory and regulatory language

- Evidence-based policy and procedures

ANA's *Nursing: Scope and Standards of Practice* (2004, p. 1) is the document defined and promoted by the profession that "describes a competent level of nursing practice and professional performance common to all registered nurses" (p.1). Each standard is an authoritative statement ". . . by which the nursing profession describes the responsibilities for which its practitioners are accountable" (ANA, 2004, p. 1) and ". . . by which the quality of practice, service, or education can be evaluated" (ANA, 2004, p. 49). Further detailing of the expected level of performance is currently represented as specific measurement criteria for each nursing process component or professional performance category. Additional refinement of each measurement criterion will be necessary to assure the language identifies a behavioral, cognitive, or motor competency required for the individual to be able to function in accordance with each standard.

See the Appendix for a summary of other organizations' statements on competency.

EVALUATING COMPETENCE

The ANA Standards of Practice and Standards of Professional Performance "are authoritative statements by which the nursing profession describes the responsibilities for which its practitioners are accountable" (ANA, 2004, p. 1). The measurement criteria included with each standard "are key indicators of competent practice for each standard. For a standard to be met, all the listed measurement criteria must be met" (ANA, 2004, p. 5). Therefore, the measurement criteria are currently used to represent the competence statements for each standard of nursing practice and of professional performance.

Competence in nursing practice must be evaluated by the individual nurse (self-assessment), nurse peers, and nurses in the roles of supervisor, coach, mentor, or preceptor. In addition, other aspects of nursing performance may be evaluated by professional colleagues and patients/clients.

Competence can be evaluated by using tools that capture objective and subjective data about the individual's knowledge base and actual performance and are appropriate for the specific situation and the desired outcome of the competence evaluation. Such tools and methods include but are not limited to: direct observation, patient records, portfolio, demonstrations, skills lab, performance evaluation, peer review, certification, credentialing, privileging, simulation exercises, computer simulated and virtual reality testing, targeted continuing education with outcomes measurement, employer skills validation and practice evaluations. However, no single evaluation tool or method can guarantee competence.

Summary: As the professional association representing the profession of over 3.1 million nurses, ANA leads the profession in addressing the complex issue of assuring professional competence of the nursing workforce.

The ANA supports the following principles in regard to competence in the nursing profession:

- Registered nurses are individually responsible and accountable for maintaining competence.

- The public has a right to expect nurses to demonstrate competence throughout their careers.

- Competence is definable, measurable, and can be evaluated.

- Context determines what competencies are necessary.

- Competence is dynamic, and both an outcome and an ongoing process.

- The nursing profession and professional organizations must shape and guide any process assuring nurse competence.

- The measurement criteria contained in the ANA's various scope and standards of practice documents are the competence statements for each standard of nursing practice and of professional performance.

- Regulatory bodies define minimal standards for regulation of practice to protect the public.

- Employers are responsible and accountable to provide an environment conducive to competent practice.

- Assurance of competence is the shared responsibility of the profession, individual nurses, regulatory bodies, employers, and other key stakeholders.

Recommendations/Next Steps

The definitions of competence and competency and the accompanying descriptions of related concepts should be included in the ANA scope and standards documents. This information should also be used to guide nursing education, staff development, credentialing, and legislative and regulatory initiatives. Dissemination can be accomplished through publication in *The American*

Nurse, American Nurse Today, www.nursingworld.org, and educational programs across the country.

Many issues and questions remain and must be addressed, including but not limited to:

- How does the work environment impact the assurance and maintenance of competence?

- How should basic competence or specialized competence be measured?

- Who pays for it?

- What are the legal issues related to the assurance and maintenance of competence?

- How will or should competency measurement be used in licensure and regulation? (Whittaker, Carson, & Smolenski, 2000)

- What are the implications of competence for nurses who practice as part of interprofessional teams?

ANA affirms its commitment to ongoing examination, discussion, and action related to these and other issues around competence of nurses.

References

American Association of Colleges of Nursing. (1998). *The Essentials of Baccalaureate Education for Professional Nursing Practice.* Washington, DC: Author.

American Nurses Association. (2000). *Continuing professional nursing competence: Nursing's agenda for the 21ˢᵗ century.* Silver Spring: Author.

American Nurses Association. (2001). *Code of ethics for nurses with interpretive statements.* Washington, DC: Nursebooks.org.

American Nurses Association. (2003). *Nursing's social policy statement, Second edition* Washington, DC: Nursebooks.org.

American Nurses Association. (2004). *Nursing: Scope and standards of practice.* Silver Spring, MD: Nursebooks.org.

Benner, P. (1982). From novice to expert. *American Journal of Nursing.* 82(3), 402-407.

Competency and Credentialing Institute (CCI). (2007). *The CCI continued competence forum: From pieces to policy.* Retrieved January 28, 2008 from http://cc-institute.org/tt07_index.aspx

Whittaker, S., Carson, W., & Smolenski, M. (2000).Assuring continued competence-policy questions and approaches: How should the profession respond? In *Online Journal of Issues in Nursing,* Retrieved February 15, 2007 from http://www.nursingworld.org/ojin/topic10/ tpc10_4.htm

Appendix.
Summary of Other Organizations' Statements

In 1999 the **Institute of Medicine (IOM)** recommended the implementation of periodic reexamination and relicensure of physicians, nurses and other health care providers based on competence and knowledge of safety practices (IOM, 1999). In *Crossing the Quality Chasm: A New Health System for the 21st Century,* the IOM cited that "There are no consistent methods for ensuring the continued competence of health professionals within the current state licensing functions or other processes" (IOM, 2001, p. 217). The IOM has identified five areas of competence for all health care providers: patient centered care, interdisciplinary team, evidence-based practice, quality improvement and informatics (IOM, 2002). These IOM areas of competence have been expanded and articulated for nursing through the Quality and Safety Education for Nurses project (Cronenwett, Sherwood, Barnsteiner, et. al., 2007; Smith, Cronenwett, Sherwood, 2007).

The **National Council of State Boards of Nursing (NCSBN)** defines competence as "the application of knowledge and the interpersonal, decision-making and psychomotor skills expected for the practice role, within the context of public health, safety and welfare" (NCSBN, 1996, p. 5). NCSBN holds that continued competence is a critical regulatory issue for Boards of Nursing.

The **American Association of Critical Care Nurses (AACN)** Synergy Model for patient care identifies nurse competencies of concern to patients, clinical units and systems. The core concept of the AACN Synergy Model is that the needs or characteristics of patients and families influence and drive the characteristics or competencies of nurses. These competencies include:

clinical judgment, advocacy and moral agency, caring practices, collaboration, systems thinking, response to diversity, facilitation of learning, and clinical inquiry (AACN, 1999).

The **Vermont Nurse Internship Project** uses Lenburg's *Competency Outcomes Performance Assessment* which includes: assessment and intervention, communication, critical thinking, human caring relationships, management, leadership, teaching, and knowledge integration skills (Lenberg, 1999). This Internship Model describes competency development to support new and transitioning nurses. The outcome builds individual and environmental capacity for professional development, successful transition and retention (Boyer, 2002).

The **Texas Board of Nurse Examiners'** *Differentiated Entry level Competencies of Graduates of Texas Nursing Program* (2002) has organized competencies according to three major roles of the nurse: Provider of Care, Coordinator of Care, and Member of Profession. Fourteen broad competency statements describe the expected behaviors of the graduate and serve as guidelines for utilization of new graduates in practice settings and the development of plans for building upon competencies (e.g., orientation programs, job descriptions, clinical ladders). The competencies are then further described in terms of "knowledge needed to achieve the competency" and related "clinical behaviors and judgments." A major difference among the competencies for the three levels of educational preparation is the target client: beginning with the individual at the LPN level and broadening to families and groups at the BSN level.

The Joint Commission requires hospitals to assess the competency of employees when hired and then regularly throughout employment. According to The Joint Commission (2007) "competence assessment is systematic and allows for a measurable assessment of the person's ability to perform required activities. Information used as part of competence assessment may include data from performance evaluations, performance improvement, and aggregate data on competence, as well as the assessment of learning needs" (p.346).

The **Competency and Credentialing Institute (2007)** convened a think tank of nursing leaders to build consensus for a process of continued competence for professional nurses that is practical, cost-effective, transferable, and a nationally accepted platform in order to ensure patient safety and quality of care for the public. Competency is valued as central to practice and will require a revamping of educational practices, information literacy, interdisciplinary teams and learnings and is influenced by policy.

In March 2006, the **Massachusetts Board of Higher Education and the Massachusetts Organization of Nurse Executives** convened a session called *Creativity and Connections: Building the Framework for the Future of Nursing Education and Practice*. One of the top priorities of the group was to develop consensus on competencies to serve as a framework for educational curriculum. The focus is on the development of a seamless continuum of nursing education built on a set of identified competencies and use of these competencies as a framework to develop a statewide transition into practice model. Nursing Core Competencies for the Nurse of the Future have been developed and the group is now seeking feedback (Massachusetts Board of Higher Education Nursing Initiative, 2007).

References

American Association of Critical Care Nurses. (1999). *The AACN Synergy Model for Patient Care*. Retrieved March 27, 2007 from http://www.certcorp.org/certcorp/certcorp.nsf/vwdoc/SynMode l

Board of Nurse Examiners for the State of Texas and the Texas Board of Vocational Nurse Examiners. (2002). *Differentiated entry level competencies of graduates of Texas nursing programs*. Available at http://sacs.utpa.edu/sacs/federaRequirements/federal4.2Resources/federal4.2R1 6_del-comp.pdf

Boyer, S. (2002). *Vermont nurse internship project—a transition to practice model*. Retrieved February 15, 2007 from www.vnip.org

Competency and Credentialing Institute (CCI). (2007). *The CCI continued competence forum: From pieces to policy*. Retrieved January 28, 2008 from http://cc-institute.org/tt07_index.aspx

Cronenwett, L., Sherwood, G., Barnsteiner, J., Disch, J., Johnson, J., Mitchell, P., et al. (2007). Quality and safety education for nurses. *Nursing Outlook, 55*(3), 122–131.

Institute of Medicine. (1999). *To err is human*. Washington, DC: National Academies Press.

Institute of Medicine. (2001). *Crossing the quality chasm*. Washington, DC: National Academy Press.

Institute of Medicine. (2002). *Who will keep the public healthy: Educating health professionals for the 21st century.* Washington, DC: National Academy Press.

Lenburg, C. (1999). The Framework, Concepts and Methods of the Competency Outcomes and Performance Assessment (COPA) Model. *Online Journal of Issues in Nursing.* Available http://www.nursingworld .org/ojin/topic10/tpc10_2.htm

Massachusetts Board of Higher Education Nursing Initiative (2007). *Creativity and connections: Building the framework for the future of nursing education and practice.* Available at http://www.mass.edu/ currentinit/currentinitNursingPublications.asp

National Council of State Boards of Nursing. (1996). *Assuring competence: A regulatory responsibility.* Chicago: Author.

Smith, E. L., Cronenwett, L., & Sherwood, G. (2007). Current assessments of quality and safety education in nursing. *Nursing Outlook, 55,* 132–127.

The Joint Commission. (2007).*Comprehensive Accreditation Manual for Hospitals: The Official Handbook.* Oakbrook Terrace, IL: Author.

APPENDIX C.

The Development of Professional Nursing and Its Foundational Documents

The American Nurses Association has long been instrumental in the development of three foundational documents for professional nursing: its code of ethics, its scope and standards of practice, and its statement of social policy. Each document contributes to further understanding the context of nursing practice at the time of publication and reflects the history of the evolution of the nursing profession in the United States.

Advancing communication technologies have expanded the revision process to permit ever-increasing numbers of registered nurses to contribute to the open dialogue and review activities. This ensures that the final published versions not only codify the consensus of the profession at the time of publication, but also reflect the experiences of those working in the profession at all levels and in all settings.

A Timeline of Development

1859 Florence Nightingale publishes Notes on Nursing: *What It Is and What It Is Not.*

1896 The Nurses' Associated Alumnae of the United States and Canada is founded. Later to become the American Nurses Association (ANA), its first purpose is to establish and maintain a code of ethics.

1940 A "Tentative Code" is published in *The American Journal of Nursing*, although never formally adopted.

1950 *Code for Professional Nurses*, in the form of 17 provisions that are a substantive revision of the "Tentative Code" of 1940, is unanimously accepted by the ANA House of Delegates.

1952 *Nursing Research* publishes its premiere issue.

1956 *Code for Professional Nurses* is amended.

1960 *Code for Professional Nurses* is revised.

1968 *Code for Professional Nurses* is substantively revised, condensing the 17 provisions of the 1960 Code into 10 provisions.

1973 ANA publishes its first *Standards of Nursing Practice*.

1976 ANA publishes *Standards of Gerontological Nursing Practice*, its first such for a nursing specialty practice.

1976 *Code for Nurses with Interpretive Statements*, a modification of the provisions and interpretive statements, is published as 11 provisions.

1980 ANA publishes Nursing: *A Social Policy Statement*.

1985 The National Institutes of Health organizes the National Center for Nursing Research.

ANA publishes *Titling for Licensure*.

Code for Nurses with Interpretive Statements retains the provisions of the 1976 version and includes revised interpretive statements.

The ANA House of Delegates forms a task force to formally document the scope of practice for nursing.

1987 ANA publishes *The Scope of Nursing Practice*.

1990   The ANA House of Delegates forms a task force to revise the 1973 *Standards of Nursing Practice.*

1991   ANA publishes *Standards of Clinical Nursing Practice.*

1995   ANA publishes *Nursing's Social Policy Statement.*

1995   The Congress of Nursing Practice directs the Committee on Nursing Practice Standards and Guidelines to establish a process for periodic review and revision of nursing standards.

1996   ANA publishes *Scope and Standards of Advanced Practice Registered Nursing.*

1998   ANA publishes *Standards of Clinical Nursing Practice, 2nd Edition* (also known as the *Clinical Standards*).

2001   *Code of Ethics for Nurses with Interpretive Statements* is accepted by the ANA House of Delegates.

ANA publishes *Bill of Rights for Registered Nurses.*

2002   ANA publishes *Nursing's Agenda for the Future: A Call to the Nation.*

2003   ANA publishes *Nursing's Social Policy Statement, 2nd Edition.*

2004   ANA publishes *Nursing: Scope and Standards of Practice.*

2008   APRN Consensus Model published by the APRN Consensus Work Group and APRN Joint Dialogue Group.

ANA publishes *Professional Role Competence Position Statement.*

ANA publishes *Specialization and Credentialing in Nursing Revisited: Understanding the Issues, Advancing the Profession.*

2010   ANA publishes *Nursing's Social Policy Statement: The Essence of the Profession.*

ANA publishes *Nursing: Scope and Standards of Practice, 2nd Edition.*

Some Specialty Nursing Practice Scope and Standards

Since 1976, the American Nurses Association has been collaborating with nursing specialty practice organizations to develop and publish first the standards of nursing practice specialties, and later to incorporate the scope of such specialty practice. (See the timeline starting on page 89.) Each of these ANA titles on the scope and standards of specialty nursing practice has been developed in conjunction with a workgroup of specialist practitioners, and often formally co-published with one or more specialty organizations.

Addictions Nursing Practice, Scope and Standards of
  Co-published with International Nurses Society on Addictions

Cardiovascular Nursing: Scope and Standards of Practice
  Co-published with American College of Cardiology Foundation, and endorsed by 13 specialty organizations

Corrections Nursing: Scope and Standards of Practice

Faith Community Nursing: Scope and Standards of Practice
  Co-published with Health Ministries Association, Inc.

Diabetes Nursing: Scope and Standards of Practice
  Co-published with American Association of Diabetes Educators

Forensic Nursing: Scope and Standards of Practice
  Co-published with International Association of Forensic Nurses (IAFN)

Genetics/Genomics Nursing: Scope and Standards of Practice
  Co-published with International Society of Nurses in Genetics (ISONG)

Gerontological Nursing: Scope and Standards of Practice
  Developed in conjunction with National Gerontological Nursing Association

HIV/AIDS Nursing: Scope and Standards of Practice
  Co-published with American Association of Nurses in AIDS Care (ANAC)

Holistic Nursing: Scope and Standards of Practice (2007)
  Co-published with American Holistic Nurses Association (AHNA)

Home Health Nursing: Scope and Standards of Practice

Hospice and Palliative Nursing: Scope and Standards of Practice
   Co-published with Hospice and Palliative Nurses Association (HPNA)

Holistic Nursing: Scope and Standards of Practice
   Co-published with American Holistic Nurses Association (AHNA)

Intellectual and Developmental Disabilities Nursing: Scope and Standards of Practice
   Co-published with Nursing Division of the American Association on Mental Retardation (AAMR; now, American Association on Intellectual and Developmental Disabilities, AAIDD)

Legal Nurse Consulting: Scope and Standards of Practice
   Co-published with American Association of Legal Nurse Consultants (AALNC)

Neonatal Nursing: Scope and Standards of Practice
   Co-published with National Association of Neonatal Nurses (NANN)

Neuroscience Nursing Practice, Scope and Standards of
   Co-published with American Association of Neuroscience Nurses (AANN)

Nursing Administration: Scope and Standards of Practice

Nursing Informatics: Scope and Standards of Practice

Nursing Professional Development: Scope and Standards of Practice
   Co-published with National Nursing Staff Development Organization (NNSDO)

Pain Management Nursing: Scope and Standards of Practice
   Co-published with American Society of Pain Management Nurses (ASPMN)

Pediatric Nursing: Scope and Standards of Practice (2008)
   Co-published with National Association of Pediatric Nurse Practitioners (NAPNAP) and International Society of Pediatric Nurses (ISPN)

Plastic Surgery Nursing: Scope and Standards of Practice
   Co-published with American Society of Plastic Surgical Nurses (ASPSN)

Psychiatric–Mental Health Nursing: Scope and Standards of Practice
   Co-published with American Psychiatric Nurses Association (APNA) and
   International Society of Psychiatric-Mental Health Nurses (ISPN)

Public Health Nursing: Scope and Standards of Practice

Radiology Nursing: Scope and Standards of Practice
   Co-published with American Radiological Nurses Association (ARNA)

School Nursing: Scope and Standards of Practice
   Co-published with National Association of School Nurses (NASN)

Transplant Nursing: Scope and Standards of Practice
   Co-published with International Transplant Nurses Society (ITNS)

Vascular Nursing Practice, Scope and Standards of
   Co-published with Society for Vascular Nursing (SVN)

Appendix D.

Nursing: Scope and Standards of Practice (2004)

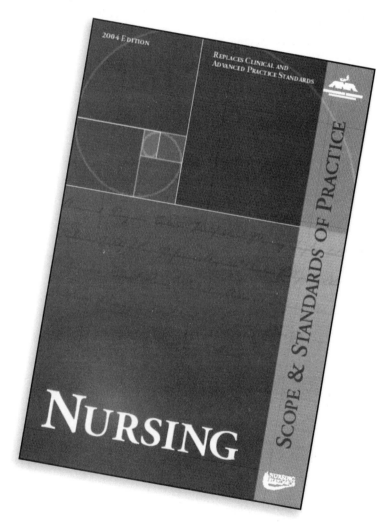

The context in this appendix is not current and is of historical significance only.

CONTENTS

These appendixes and the index are not included in this reproduction.

PREFACE

The authority for the practice of nursing is based on a social contract that acknowledges the professional rights and responsibilities of nursing and includes mechanisms for public accountability. *Nursing's Social Policy Statement* (ANA, 2003) identifies that "nursing is the protection, promotion, and optimization of health and abilities, prevention of illness and injury, alleviation of suffering through the diagnosis and treatment of human response, and advocacy in the care of individuals, families, communities, and populations."

Nursing: Scope and Standards of Practice outlines the expectations of the professional role within which all registered nurses must practice. This scope statement and these updated standards of nursing practice guide, define, and direct professional nursing practice in all settings. *Nursing: Scope and Standards of Practice* is to be used in conjunction with *Nursing's Social Policy Statement* (ANA, 2003) and the *Code of Ethics for Nurses with Interpretive Statements* (ANA, 2001). These three resources provide a complete and definitive description for better understanding by specialty nursing organizations, policy makers, and the public of nursing practice and nursing's accountability to the public in the United States.

Development of Scope and Standards of Nursing Practice

The American Nurses Association (ANA) has actively engaged in scope of practice and standards development initiatives since the late 1960s. ANA published the first *Standards of Nursing Practice* for the nursing profession in 1973. The standards were generic in nature and focused on the basic nursing process—a critical thinking model applicable to all registered nurses—comprised of assessment, diagnosis, planning, implementation, and evaluation.

Over the years, specialty nursing organizations also have developed scope of practice statements and standards of practice for those registered nurses engaged in specialty practice, such as addictions, gerontology, pediatrics, hospice and palliative care, developmental disabilities, rehabilitation, psychiatric-mental health, oncology, nursing administration, informatics, professional development, and others. Some of these scopes and standards of practice were developed in collaboration with ANA; others were developed separately. Thus, the various scope and standards documents sometimes differed widely in purpose, scope, and format, and were limited in their ability to support an integrated picture of nursing and its contributions to health care.

In 1990, the ANA House of Delegates charged a task force to define the nature and purpose of standards of practice for nursing. The task force's report included a recommendation that the 1973 *Standards of Nursing Practice* be revised. A participative process was instituted that permitted incorporation of broad input and comments from state nurses associations and specialty nursing organizations.

In 1991, after a long and fruitful collaboration with specialty nursing organizations, ANA published *Standards of Clinical Nursing Practice (Clinical Standards)*. These professional clinical practice and performance standards established a common language and consistent format to clarify and strengthen nursing's ability to define the actual conduct of nursing practice within all practice areas. This initiative also established a framework within which specialty organizations and the ANA could work together to develop standards that foster a collaborative approach to decision-making concerning the practice of nursing. Throughout the 1990s, these standards significantly shaped nursing practice, served as a model for regulatory language, and provided a framework for other important works such as *Scope and Standards of Advanced Practice Registered Nursing* (ANA, 1996).

In 1995, the ANA Congress of Nursing Practice charged the Committee on Nursing Practice Standards and Guidelines with establishing a process for periodic review and revision, when necessary, of the standards documents. The process used in the development of the 1998 *Standards of Clinical Nursing Practice, 2nd Edition*, incorporated input from major stakeholders by:

(1) An assessment of the congruency of *Clinical Standards* with other contemporary ANA documents, e.g., *Nursing's Social Policy Statement* and the Code of Ethics;

(2) A survey of individual registered nurses as to their perceptions of the frequency of use and relevancy of *Clinical Standards* to their practice; and

(3) A survey of specialty nursing organizations as to the usefulness of *Clinical Standards* in regulatory and legislative activities.

Registered nurses throughout the country responded and affirmed the importance and usefulness of the original *Standards of Clinical Nursing Practice*.

In 2001, the Congress on Nursing Practice and Economics (CNPE) called for the establishment of a workgroup to conduct the review of *Standards of Clinical Nursing Practice, 2nd Edition*. The workgroup was assigned the task of incorporating into the new document the standards of practice for professional registered nurses, advanced practice registered nurses, and nurses in role specialties. Additional responsibilities included developing a corresponding contemporary statement of the scope of nursing practice.

The 2004 *Nursing: Scope and Standards of Practice* underwent a review process similar to the one implemented for the 1998 *Clinical Standards* with the significant addition of the opportunity for electronic web-based review that allowed individual comments. The CNPE workgroup:

- conducted an assessment for congruency of the new Scope and Standards with other ANA documents,

- distributed a working draft of the document to attendees of the 2002 ANA Convention,

- conducted a focus group at the 2002 ANA Convention,

- notified ANA's constituent member associations and the specialty nursing organizations that input was being requested on the draft document, and

- posted the draft document on ANA's www.NursingWorld.org web site for public review and comment by interested nurses and others.

All comments and suggestions were reviewed and considered by the workgroup in preparing this document. Reviews by the ANA Congress on Nursing Practice and Economics Committee on Clinical Practice Standards and Guidelines and the Congress on Nursing Practice and Economics culminated in the final edits of *Nursing: Scope and Standards of Practice*.

As with previous versions of this document, the real work begins now. The profession must incorporate the written word into practice settings across the country. The goal is to improve the health and well-being of all individuals, communities, and populations through the significant and visible contributions of registered nurses utilizing standards-based practice.

$$\cdot \cdot \cdot \cdot \cdot$$

Additional Content

To provide context for the development of Nursing: Scope and Standards of Practice (2004), the content of these appendices have been indexed:

- Appendix A: Timeline of the Development of Foundational Nursing Documents
- Appendix B: *Standards of Nursing Practice* (1973)
- Appendix C: *The Scope of Nursing Practice* (1987)
- Appendix D: *Standards of Clinical Nursing Practice* (1991)
- Appendix E: *Standards of Clinical Nursing Practice, 2nd Edition* (1998)
- Appendix F: *Scope and Standards of Advanced Practice Registered Nursing,* (1996)
- Appendix G: Scope and Standards Contributors, 1973–1998.

INTRODUCTION

Function of the Scope of Practice Statement

The scope of practice statement describes the *who, what, where, when, why,* and *how* of nursing practice. Each of these questions must be sufficiently answered to provide a complete picture of the practice and its boundaries and membership. The profession of nursing has one scope of practice that encompasses the full range of nursing practice. The depth and breadth in which individual registered nurses engage in the total scope of nursing practice is dependent upon education, experience, role, and the population served.

Function of Standards

Standards are authoritative statements by which the nursing profession describes the responsibilities for which its practitioners are accountable. Consequently, standards reflect the values and priorities of the profession. Standards provide direction for professional nursing practice and a framework for the evaluation of this practice. Written in measurable terms, standards also define the nursing profession's accountability to the public and the outcomes for which registered nurses are responsible.

Development of Standards

A professional nursing organization has a responsibility to its members and to the public it serves to develop standards of practice. Standards of professional nursing practice may pertain to general or specialty practice. As the professional organization for all registered nurses, the American Nurses Association (ANA) has assumed the responsibility for developing generic standards that apply to the practice of all professional nurses. Standards do, however, belong to the profession and, thus, require broad input into their development and revision. *Nursing: Scope and Standards of Practice* (*Scope and Standards*) describes a competent level of nursing practice and professional performance common to all registered nurses.

Assumptions

1. *A link exists between the professional work environment and the registered nurse's ability to practice.*

Nursing: Scope and Standards of Practice focuses primarily on the processes involved in the conduct of nursing practice and the performance of professional role activities. Although these standards apply to all registered nurses in all areas of practice, it is recognized that there is tremendous variability in these environments and practice settings. Recognizing the link between the professional work environment and the nurse's ability to practice, employers must provide an environment that supports nursing practice and decision-making.

2. *Nursing practice is individualized.*

The second assumption is that nursing practice is individualized to meet the unique needs of the patient or situation. This includes respect for the patient's and family's or support system's goals and preferences regarding care. Given that one of the registered nurse's primary responsibilities is education, nurses provide patients, colleagues, and others with appropriate information to make informed decisions regarding health care and healthcare issues, including health promotion, prevention of disease, and attainment of a dignified and peaceful death.

3. *Nurses establish partnerships.*

The third assumption is that the registered nurse establishes a partnership with the patient, family, support system, and other healthcare providers. In this partnership, the nurse works collaboratively to coordinate the care provided to the patient. The degree of participation by the patient, family, support system, and other healthcare providers will vary based upon needs, preferences, and abilities.

Organizing Principles

Nursing: Scope and Standards of Practice uses the term *patient* to include individuals, families, groups, communities, and populations to whom the registered nurse is providing services as sanctioned by the state nurse practice acts. The cultural, racial, and ethnic diversity of the patient must always be taken into account in providing nursing services.

Scope and Standards is generic in nature and applies to all professional registered nurses engaged in practice, regardless of clinical or functional specialty, practice setting, or educational preparation. When defining expectations associated with their particular area of specialty nursing practice, professional nursing organizations and groups may elect to develop more tailored and detailed scope of practice statements, standards, and associated measurement criteria built on the framework provided in *Nursing: Scope and Standards of Practice*.

The Standards of Nursing Practice content consists of Standards of Practice and Standards of Professional Performance, which include the following:

Standards of Practice

1 Assessment
2 Diagnosis
3 Outcomes Identification
4 Planning
5 Implementation
   5a Coordination of Care
   5b Health Teaching and Health Promotion
   5c Consultation
   5d Prescriptive Authority
6 Evaluation

Standards of Professional Practice

7 Quality of Practice
8 Education
9 Professional Practice Evaluation
10 Collegiality
11 Collaboration
12 Ethics
13 Research
14 Resource Utilization
15 Leadership

Standards of Practice

The six Standards of Practice describe a competent level of nursing care as demonstrated by the critical thinking model known as the nursing process. The nursing process includes the components of assessment, diagnosis, outcomes identification, planning, implementation, and evaluation. The nursing process encompasses all significant actions taken by registered nurses, and forms the foundation of the nurse's decision-making.

Several themes span all areas of nursing practice, are fundamental to many of the standards, and have emerged as being consistently and significantly influential in current nursing practice. These themes include:

- Providing age-appropriate and culturally and ethnically sensitive care
- Maintaining a safe environment
- Educating patients about healthy practices and treatment modalities
- Assuring continuity of care
- Coordinating the care across settings and among caregivers
- Managing information
- Communicating effectively
- Utilizing technology

These highlighted themes are reflected in the measurement criteria, although the wording may differ among the various standards. With future revisions of *Scope and Standards*, some of these themes may evolve into new standard statements.

Standards of Professional Performance

The nine Standards of Professional Performance describe a competent level of behavior in the professional role—including activities related to quality of practice, education, professional practice evaluation, collegiality, collaboration, ethics, research, resource utilization, and leadership. The last standard is new in this revision and addresses the leadership required of registered nurses in their practice. All registered nurses are expected to engage in professional role activities, including leadership, appropriate to their education and position. Registered nurses are accountable for their professional actions to themselves, their patients, their peers, and, ultimately, to society.

Measurement Criteria

Measurement criteria are key indicators of competent practice for each standard. *Nursing: Scope and Standards of Practice* includes criteria that allow the standards to be measured. For a standard to be met, all the listed measurement criteria must be met.

Standards should remain stable over time, as they reflect the philosophical values of the profession. Measurement criteria, however, can be revised more frequently to incorporate advancements in scientific knowledge and expectations for nursing practice. Additional measurement criteria that are applicable only to advanced practice registered nurses, or to those in nursing role specialties, are included for select standards of practice and professional performance.

In this document, words such as *appropriate* and *possible* are sometimes used. A document of this kind cannot account for all potential scenarios that the professional registered nurse might encounter in practice. The registered nurse will need to exercise judgment based on education and experience in determining what is appropriate or possible for a patient or in a particular situation. Further direction may be available from documents such as guidelines for practice or agency standards, policies, procedures, and protocols.

Relationship to Guidelines

Guidelines describe a process of patient care management, which has the potential for improving the quality of clinical and patient decision-making. As systematically developed statements based on available scientific evidence and expert opinion, practice guidelines address the care of specific patient populations or phenomena, whereas standards provide a broad framework for practice.

Summary

Nursing: Scope and Standards of Practice delineates the professional responsibilities of all professional registered nurses engaged in nursing practice, regardless of setting. *Scope and Standards* and available nursing practice guidelines can serve as a basis for:

- Quality improvement systems

- Data bases

- Regulatory systems

- Healthcare reimbursement and financing methodologies

- Development and evaluation of nursing service delivery systems and organizational structures

- Certification activities

- Position descriptions and performance appraisals

- Agency policies, procedures, and protocols

- Educational offerings

To best serve the public's health and the nursing profession, nursing must continue in its efforts to develop standards of practice and guidelines for practice. Nursing must also examine how standards and practice guidelines can be disseminated and used most effectively to enhance and promote the quality of practice. In addition, standards and practice guidelines must be evaluated on an ongoing basis, with revisions made as necessary. The dynamic nature of the healthcare environment and the growing body of nursing research provide both the impetus and the opportunity for nursing to ensure competent nursing practice in all settings for all patients and to promote ongoing professional development that enhances the quality of nursing practice.

SCOPE OF NURSING PRACTICE

Definition of Nursing

Nursing's Social Policy Statement, Second Edition (2003) builds on previous work and provides the following contemporary definition of nursing:

> Nursing is the protection, promotion, and optimization of health and abilities, prevention of illness and injury, alleviation of suffering through the diagnosis and treatment of human response, and advocacy in the care of individuals, families, communities, and populations.

This definition serves as the foundation for the following expanded content that describes the scope and standards of nursing practice.

Evolution of Nursing Practice

Contemporary nursing practice has its historical roots in the poorhouses, the battlefields, and the industrial revolutions in Europe and America. Initially nurses trained in hospital-based nursing schools and were employed mainly in private duty, providing care to patients in their homes. Florence Nightingale provided a foundation for nursing and the basis for autonomous nursing practice as distinctly different from medicine. Nightingale also is credited for identifying the importance of collecting empirical evidence, the underpinning of nursing's current emphasis on evidence-based practice, "What you want are facts, not opinions… The most important practical lesson that can be given to nurses is to teach them what to observe – how to observe – what symptoms indicate improvement – which are of none – which are the evidence of neglect – and what kind of neglect." (Nightingale, 1859, p. 105)

Although Nightingale recommended clinical nursing research in the mid 1800s, nurses did not follow her advice for more than 100 years. Nursing research was able to develop only as nurses received advanced educational preparation. In the early 1900s nurses received their advanced degrees in nursing education, which resulted in studies about nurses and nursing education. However, case studies on nursing interventions were conducted in the 1920s and 1930s, and the results published in the *American Journal of Nursing.*

Then in the 1950s, interest in nursing care studies began to arise. In 1952, the first issue of *Nursing Research* was published. In the 1960s, nursing studies began to explore theoretical and conceptual frameworks as a basis for practice. By the 1970s more doctorally prepared nurses were conducting research, and there was a shift to studies that focused on practice-related research and the improvement of patient care. By the 1980s there were more qualified nurse researchers than ever before, as well as an increasing availability of computers for collection and analysis of data. In 1985 the National Center for Nursing Research was established within the National Institutes of Health, putting nursing research into the mainstream of health research activities. (Grant and Massey, 1999)

In both World Wars, nurses responded to America's need for nurses to help care for the armed forces. In fact, by 1946, 31% of professional nurses had served with the troops. With advances in medical treatment and healthcare technology over the next sixty years, nurses in hospitals developed specialized nursing skills in both old and new areas of practice—medical–surgical nursing, pediatrics, anesthesia, midwifery, emergency care, mental health, critical care, neonatal care, and primary care. Nurses also increasingly engaged in addressing the need for public health interventions with at-risk communities and vulnerable populations; public health nursing was developed under its pioneer, Lillian Wald, at the Henry Street Settlement House in New York City.

During the last 50 years, nurse researchers (1950s) and nurse theorists (1960s and 1970s) greatly contributed to the expanding body of nursing knowledge with their studies of nursing practice and the development of nursing models and theories. These conceptual models and theories borrow from or share with other disciplines such as sociology, psychology, biology, and physics. For example, the work of Neuman and King built heavily on systems theory. There is also Levine's conservation model, Roger's science of unitary human beings, Roy's adaptation model, Orem's self-care model, Peplau's interpersonal relations model, and Watson's theory of caring. The 1980s brought revisions to these theories, as well as additional theories developed by nursing leaders, such as Johnson, Parse, and Leininger, that added to the theoretical thinking in nursing (George, 2002). In the 1990s, research studies tested and expanded these theories, which in turn continued to define and develop the discipline of nursing.

As nursing continued to evolve, four distinctly different advanced practice nursing groups developed to meet the increasingly complex needs of patients: clinical nurse specialist, nurse practitioner, certified nurse midwife, and certified registered nurse anesthetist. State laws and regulations have recognized and authorized the independent practice of nursing, encouraging greater numbers of registered nurses to pursue entrepreneurial activities, including establishing their own private practices. Similarly, the evolving healthcare delivery system has also provided exciting opportunities for registered nurses to move into other new roles.

Registered nurses throughout the decades have been social and political leaders and advocates, addressing many societal issues related to patient care, health, and wellness. Such issues have included protective labor laws, minimum wage, communicable disease programs, immunizations, well-baby/childcare, women's health, violence, reproductive health, end-of-life care, universal health care, social security, Medicare and Medicaid, the financing and reimbursement of health care, healthcare reform, ethics, mental health parity, confidentiality, workplace safety, and patients' rights.

Nursing has evolved into a profession with a distinct body of knowledge, university-based education, specialized practice, standards of practice, a social contract (*Nursing's Social Policy Statement,* 2003), and an ethical code (*Code of Ethics for Nurses with Interpretative Statements,* 2001). Registered nurses are concerned about the availability and accessibility of nursing care to patients, families, communities and populations. Registered nurses and the profession seek to ensure the integrity of nursing practice in all current and future healthcare systems.

The federal government collects data elements about the nursing workforce, the largest healthcare professional group in the U.S., as part of its numerous and disparate data collection activities. The most frequently cited consolidated source is the National Sample Survey of Registered Nurses (NSSRN), a sample survey of approximately 37,000 actively licensed registered nurses. The most recent National Sample Survey of Registered Nurses, conducted in March 2000 (U.S. HHS, 2002), identified that the estimated 2.7 million registered nurses are predominantly female and have an average age of 45.2 years. Increasing numbers of men are entering the profession and are estimated to number 147,000 or 5.4%. Hospitals, public/community health settings, ambulatory care settings and nursing homes/extended care continue to be the major employers of registered nurses. Although hospitals remain the primary employers, significant shifts to other settings are reflected by an increase since 1980 of 155% of registered nurses (RNs) employed in public health and community health settings and of 127% in ambulatory care settings. The number of registered nurses employed in nursing education has shown little change in the past two decades, despite a modest upward increase in the number of enrolled nursing students. A recent trend is the increased interest in nursing as a profession, prompting other professionals to change careers and enroll as second degree students in nursing education programs.

Integrating the Science and Art of Nursing

Nursing is a learned profession built upon a core body of knowledge reflective of its dual components of science and art. Nursing requires judgment and skill based upon principles of the biological, physical, behavioral, and social sciences. Nursing is a scientific discipline as well as a profession. Registered nurses employ critical thinking to integrate objective data with knowledge gained from an assessment of the subjective experiences of patients and groups. Registered nurses use this critical thinking process to apply the best available evidence and research data to the processes of diagnosis and treatment. Nurses continually evaluate quality and effectiveness of nursing practice and seek to optimize outcomes.

Nursing focuses on the promotion and maintenance of health and the prevention or resolution of disease, illness, or disability without restriction to a problem-focused orientation. The nursing needs of human beings are identified from a holistic perspective and are met within the context of a culturally sensitive, caring interpersonal relationship. Nursing includes the diagnosis and treatment of human responses to actual or potential health problems. Registered nurses employ practices that are restorative, supportive, and promotive in nature. *Restorative practices* modify the impact of illness or disease. *Supportive practices* are oriented toward modification of relationships or the environment to support health. *Promotive practices* mobilize healthy patterns of living, foster personal and family development, and support self-defined goals of individuals, families, communities, and populations.

Nursing is responsive to the changing needs of society and the expanding knowledge base of its theoretical and scientific domains. One of nursing's objectives is to achieve positive patient outcomes that maximize one's quality of life across the entire life-span. Registered nurses facilitate the interdisciplinary and comprehensive care provided by healthcare professionals, paraprofessionals, and volunteers. In other instances, nurses engage in consultation with other colleagues to inform decision-making and planning to meet patient care needs. Registered nurses often participate in interdisciplinary teams, where the overlapping skills complement each member's individual efforts.

All nursing practice, regardless of specialty, role, or setting, is fundamentally independent practice. Registered nurses are accountable for judgments made and actions taken in the course of their nursing practice. Therefore, the registered nurse is responsible for assessing individual competence and is committed to the process of lifelong learning. Registered nurses develop and maintain current knowledge and skills through formal and continuing education, and seek certification when available in their areas of practice. As independent practitioners, registered nurses are individually accountable for all aspects of their practice.

Registered nurses are bound by a professional code of ethics (*Code of Ethics for Nurses with Interpretive Statements*, 2001) and regulate themselves as individuals through peer review of practice. Peer review is a collegial process by which registered nurses are held accountable for practice. Peer evaluation fosters the refinement of knowledge, skills, and clinical decision-making at all levels and in all areas of clinical practice. Self-regulation by the profession of nursing assures quality of performance, which is the heart of the profession's social contract between the profession of nursing and society (*Nursing's Social Policy Statement*, 2003).

Registered nurses and members of various professions exchange knowledge and ideas about how to deliver high quality health care, resulting in overlaps and constantly changing professional practice boundaries. This multidisciplinary team collaboration among healthcare professionals involves recognition of the expertise of others within and outside one's profession and referral to those providers when appropriate. Such collaboration also involves some shared functions and a common focus on the same overall mission. By necessity, nursing's scope of practice has flexible boundaries.

Nursing practice is differentiated according to the registered nurse's educational preparation and level of practice, and is further defined by the role of the nurse and the work setting. Within each type of practice, individual nurses demonstrate competence along a continuum from novice to expert (Benner, 1982). Registered nurses can choose to develop expertise in a particular specialty and have this specialized knowledge base acknowledged through credentialing, such as certification or other mechanisms. Although advanced practice registered nurses continue to perform many of the same activities and interventions used by other nurses, the difference in their practice relates to a greater depth and breadth of knowledge, a greater degree of synthesis of data, and the increased complexity of skills and interventions.

Registered nurses regularly evaluate safety, effectiveness, and cost in the planning and delivery of nursing care. Nurses recognize that resources are limited and unequally distributed. As members of a profession, registered nurses work toward more equitable distribution and availability of healthcare services throughout the nation and the world.

The science of nursing is based on a critical thinking framework, known as the *nursing process*, composed of assessment, diagnosis, outcomes identification, planning, implementation, and evaluation. These steps serve as the foundation of clinical decision-making and are used to provide evidence-based practice. Wherever they practice, registered nurses use critical thinking to respond to the needs of the populations served, and use strategies that support optimal outcomes most appropriate to the patient or situation, being mindful of resource utilization.

Nursing is guided by standards of practice and standards of professional performance. *Standards* are authoritative statements by which the nursing profession describes the responsibilities for which its practitioners are accountable. Standards reflect the values and priorities of the profession and are based on research and knowledge from nursing and various other sciences and disciplines. Standards provide direction for professional nursing practice and a framework for the evaluation and improvement of practice. These ongoing assessments and evaluations are in keeping with nursing's commitment to lifelong learning, and to providing creative, deliberate, holistic, and up-to-date comprehensive care.

The art of nursing is based on a framework of caring and respect for human dignity. A compassionate approach to patient care carries a mandate to provide that care competently. Competent care is provided and accomplished through independent practice and collaborative partnerships. Collaboration may be with other colleagues or the individuals seeking support or assistance with their healthcare needs.

The art of nursing embraces dynamic processes that affect the human person including, for example, spirituality, healing, empathy, mutual respect, and compassion. These intangible aspects foster health. Nursing embraces healing. Healing is fostered by compassion, helping, listening, mentoring, coaching, teaching, exploring, being present, supporting, touching, intuition, empathy, service, cultural competence, tolerance, acceptance, nurturing, mutually creating, and conflict resolution.

The Professional Registered Nurse

A registered nurse (RN) is licensed and authorized by a state, commonwealth, or territory to practice nursing. Professional licensure of the healthcare professions was established to protect the public safety and authorize the practice of the profession. Requirements for authorization of nursing practice and the performance of certain professional nursing roles vary from jurisdiction to jurisdiction. The registered nurse's experience, education, knowledge, and abilities establish a level of competence.

The registered nurse is educationally prepared for competent practice at the beginning level upon graduation from an approved school of nursing (diploma, associate, baccalaureate, generic master's, or doctorate degree) and qualified by national examination for RN licensure. See Figure 1. Since 1965, the ANA has consistently affirmed the baccalaureate degree in nursing as the preferred educational preparation for entry into nursing practice.

Figure 1. *Educational Path to Become a Registered Nurse*

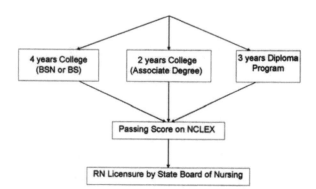

The registered nurse is educated in the art and science of nursing, with the goal of helping individuals and groups attain, maintain, and restore health whenever possible. Experienced nurses have become proficient in one or more practice areas or roles. These nurses may focus on patient care in clinical nursing practice specialties. Others function in roles that influence nursing and support the direct care rendered to patients by those professional nurses in clinical practice. Such specialized knowledge and experience may be acknowledged through an identified credentialing process. Credentialing organizations may mandate specific nursing educational requirements, as well as timely demonstrations of knowledge and experience in specialty practice.

Registered nurses may elect to pursue advanced academic studies to prepare for specialization in practice. Educational requirements vary by specialty and educational facility and may include completion of a national certification examination. See Figure 2. New models for educational preparation are evolving in response to the changing healthcare, education, and regulatory environments.

Figure 2. *Professional Specialization for Registered Nurses*

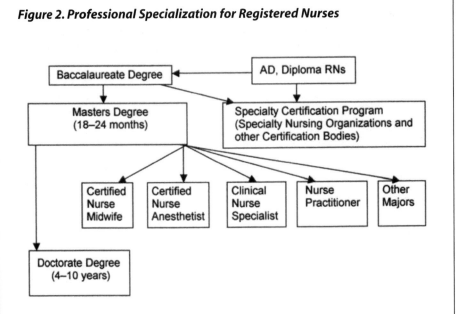

Advanced Practice Registered Nurses

Advanced practice registered nurses are RNs who have acquired advanced specialized clinical knowledge and skills to provide health care. These nurses are expected to hold a masters or doctorate degree. They build on the practice of registered nurses by demonstrating a greater depth and breadth of knowledge, a greater synthesis of data, increased complexity of skills and interventions, and significant role autonomy. As within all nursing practice, the level of expertise of the advanced practice registered nurse increases as they journey from novice to expert (Benner, 1982).

Advanced practice registered nurse (APRN) is the umbrella term used to identify the advanced practice roles of certified registered nurse anesthetist, certified nurse midwife, clinical nurse specialist, and nurse practitioner. Although the scope of practice for each of these advanced practice registered nurses is distinguishable from the others, there is an overlapping of knowledge and skills within these roles. The following descriptions are illustrative of these roles and not an exhaustive delineation of function.

Certified Registered Nurse Anesthetist: Certified registered nurse anesthetists (CRNAs) are graduates of nurse anesthesia educational programs accredited by the Council on Accreditation of Nurse Anesthesia Educational Programs or its predecessor, and have passed the certification examination administered by the Council on Certification of Nurse Anesthetists or its predecessor. CRNAs provide anesthesia and anesthesia-related care in the following domains: (1) the performance of pre-anesthetic preparation and evaluation; (2) anesthesia induction, maintenance, and emergence, including administration of appropriate drugs and techniques and local, regional, and general anesthesia, and the establishment of invasive monitoring; (3) post-anesthesia care; (4) acute and chronic pain management; and (5) associated clinical support functions, such as respiratory care and emergency resuscitation.

Certified Nurse-Midwife: Certified nurse-midwives (CNMs) are registered nurses, educated in the two disciplines of nursing and midwifery, who possess evidence of certification according to the requirements of the American College of Nurse-Midwives. Midwifery practice conducted by CNMs is the independent management of women's health care, including prescriptive authority. This practice focuses particularly on pregnancy, childbirth, the postpartum period, care of the newborn, and the family planning and gynecological needs of women. CNMs practice within a healthcare system that provides for consultation, collaborative management, or referral as indicated by the health status of the patient.

Clinical Nurse Specialist: Clinical nurse specialists (CNSs) are registered nurses, who have graduate level nursing preparation at the master's or doctoral level as a CNS. They are clinical experts in evidence-based nursing practice within a specialty area, treating and managing the health concerns of patients and populations. The CNS specialty may be focused on individuals, populations, settings, type of care, type of problem, or diagnostic systems subspecialty. CNSs practice autonomously and integrate knowledge of disease and medical treatments into the assessment, diagnosis, and treatment of patients' illnesses. These nurses design, implement, and evaluate both patient-specific and population-based programs of care. CNSs provide leadership in advancing the practice of nursing to achieve quality and cost-effective patient outcomes as well as provide leadership of multidisciplinary groups in designing and implementing innovative alternative solutions that address system problems and/or patient care issues. In many jurisdictions, CNSs, as direct care providers, perform comprehensive health assessments, develop differential diagnoses, and may have prescriptive authority. Prescriptive authority allows them to provide pharmacologic and nonpharmacologic treatments and order diagnostic and laboratory tests in addressing and managing specialty health problems of patients and populations. CNSs serve as patient advocates, consultants, and researchers in various settings.

Nurse Practitioner: Nurse practitioners (NPs) are registered nurses who have graduate level nursing preparation at the master's or doctoral level as a nurse practitioner. NPs perform comprehensive assessments and promote health and the prevention of illness and injury. These advanced practice registered nurses diagnose; develop differential diagnoses; order, conduct, supervise, and interpret diagnostic and laboratory tests; and prescribe pharmacologic and non-pharmacologic treatments in the direct management of acute and chronic illness and disease. Nurse practitioners provide health and medical care in primary, acute, and long-term care settings. NPs may specialize in areas such as family, geriatric, pediatric, primary, or acute care. Nurse practitioners practice autonomously and in collaboration with other healthcare professionals to treat and manage patients' health problems, and serve in various settings as researchers, consultants, and patient advocates for individuals, families, groups, and communities.

Registered Nurses in Role Specialties

As identified in *Nursing's Social Policy Statement, 2nd Edition* (2003), continuation of the profession is dependent on the education of nurses, appropriate organization of nursing services, continued expansion of nursing knowledge, and the development and adoption of policies. Such initiatives demand that registered nurses be adequately prepared for nursing role specialties, (those advanced levels of nursing practice that intersect with another body of knowledge), have a direct influence on nursing practice, and support the delivery of direct care rendered to patients by other registered nurses. Examples of nursing role specialty practice areas include administration, education, professional development, informatics, case management, quality initiatives, publishing, law, and research. Registered nurses in such role specialties generally hold master's or doctoral degrees. A registered nurse may enter a role specialty as a novice with goals to achieve the necessary education and experience for this type of advanced practice.

Settings for Nursing Practice

Nursing practice occurs whenever and wherever a registered nurse interacts with a patient, family, or group of persons, who experience or desire a change in their level of physical, mental, emotional, environmental, or spiritual well-being, or when the maintenance of their current level of well-being requires nursing action(s). The practice settings for the delivery of nursing care are continuously changing in response to the dynamic nature of today's healthcare environment. Settings may include, but are not limited to, academic medical centers, ambulatory health centers, clinics, communities, homes, hospices, hospitals, physician offices, and schools. In addition, nurses may practice in settings such as community nursing organizations, work sites, corporate offices, managed care organizations, correctional facilities, entrepreneurial private practices, pharmaceutical companies, professional nursing and healthcare organizations, and universities and colleges.

Registered nurses use telehealth technology in the delivery of nursing services in healthcare facilities, clinics, private offices, and the home. Nursing practice also occurs when nursing services are requested on behalf of a patient, such as a request for a consultation, or when registered nurses advocate for care that promotes health and prevents disease, illness, or disability for individuals or communities. Nurses through employment or voluntary participation, influence civic activities and the regulatory, and legislative arena at the local, state, national, or international level.

Continued Commitment to the Profession

Nursing is a dynamic profession, blending evidence-based practice with intuition, caring, and compassion to provide quality care. The nursing profession contracts with society to promote health, to do no harm, and to respond with skill and caring when change, birth, illness, disease, or death is experienced. Care is provided without regard to a person's background, identity, race, creed, circumstances, or religion.

Patients give nurses permission to enter their lives and share their most intimate life experiences. Registered nurses remain in nursing to promote, advocate for, and strive to protect the health, safety, and rights of those patients, families, communities, and populations. Registered nurses value their roles as advocates in dealing with barriers encountered in obtaining health care. Similarly, society values nursing care that resolves problems or manages health promoting behaviors (*Nursing's Social Policy Statement, 2003*).

Registered nurses experience rewarding challenges and opportunities in health care focusing on care of the whole person with various physical, psychological, and environmental needs and stressors. This involves commitment to help patients improve their physical and mental health, enrich their quality of life, reduce personal and environmental risks, and prevent disease, illness, and disability. Registered nurses prepare themselves to be resourceful, to respond to the challenges of delivering nursing care to individuals and communities, to incorporate technology into their art of caring, and to remain visionaries as the future unfolds.

Nursing also strives to strengthen individual practice through accountability and continued learning. Registered nurses seek to advance the profession through active involvement in civic activities, membership and support of professional associations, collective bargaining, and workplace advocacy. The registered nurse who articulates the goals, values, and integrity of nursing as described in *Code of Ethics for Nurses with Interpretive Statements* (ANA, 2001) ensures both nursing's commitment to the society it serves and the growth and progress of nursing itself. Registered nurses reflect these values in every day nursing practice through mentoring, listening, coaching, teaching, conflict resolution, and respecting diversity. The nurse owes the same duties to self as to others, including the responsibility to preserve professional integrity and safety, to maintain competence, and to continue personal and professional growth (ANA, 2001).

Nursing is an integral part of health care, and is indispensable to the functioning of the healthcare system. Registered nurses, as the largest group of healthcare professionals, utilize the power of their profession to make a positive impact on healthcare services and delivery. Nurses identify and champion the healthcare needs of the population, promote a safe environment, steward healthcare resources and promote universal access to healthcare services.

Professional Trends and Issues

Healthcare costs continue to escalate, prompting renewed calls for healthcare reform. Individuals and families face greater healthcare insurance premiums and deductibles as employers and insurance entities decrease their payment share for the same or, often lesser, coverage. Increasing numbers of uninsured persons join many of those with healthcare benefits in deferring preventive health and dental care and only seeking healthcare services for acute illness or injury. Self treatment and reliance on complementary and alternative therapies continue to garner an increasing market share as individuals become more involved in their own care and seek new ways to achieve health.

Today, as in the past, nursing remains pivotal to improving the health status of the public and ensuring safe, effective, quality care. Registered nurses provide a critical safety net in health care, but have been consistently invisible in the practice and reimbursement environments. Nursing care activities have not been identified by unique coding systems that would allow billing as direct services. Research continues to demonstrate and reaffirm that effective nursing care from registered nurses prevents adverse patient outcomes (Aiken et al, 2002). Although the evidence of nursing's contribution and its monetary value to health care is slowly being recognized, the current shortage of registered nurses compounds the issue and must be addressed from both the supply and demand perspectives.

The American Nurses Association and more than 100 specialty nursing organizations are identifying key initiatives and generating solutions to counter the nursing shortage, which is the major issue that needs to be addressed by the profession, healthcare industry, and government in the next decade (ANA, 2002). Nursing shortages have occurred cyclically throughout the last century. Unfortunately, the problems associated with an increasingly difficult healthcare work environment (control over the practice environment, staffing levels, mandatory overtime, salaries and benefits, availability of ancillary and technical supports, and access to staff development and education), as well as the burdensome structure of the healthcare system, have not been adequately addressed.

Currently, registered nurses and nurse faculty match the demographics of our aging population (National Sample Survey of Registered Nurses, March 2000; U.S. HHS, 2002). The adequate supply of registered nurses in clinical practice settings can only be replenished and supplemented if sufficient numbers of students enroll in nursing education programs that are supported with appropriate numbers of available teaching faculty. However, the nursing faculty shortage is projected to worsen in the next few years with the anticipated retirements of the aging faculty. Experienced registered nurses elect to remain in clinical settings or move to other healthcare venues, rather than suffer pay cuts associated with today's low faculty salaries. With faculty departing for retirement, a secondary consequence of significant magnitude will be a decline in research and publications so necessary for generating nursing knowledge.

Registered nurses must proactively deal with constant change and must be prepared for an evolving healthcare environment that includes advanced technologies. The incorporation of technologies, however, is not without risk, and demands due diligence by registered nurses to consider the impact on the scope of nursing practice and the ethical implications for healthcare consumers, as well as for the nurse.

The healthcare industry has been challenged to improve patient safety, both patient and practitioner satisfaction, patient outcomes, and the profitability of the healthcare organization (Kennedy, 2003). In 1999, the Institute of Medicine (IOM) described the nation's healthcare system as fractured, prone to errors, and detrimental to safe patient care (IOM, 1999). The IOM has identified six aims for improvement so that the healthcare system is: safe, effective, patient-centered, timely, efficient, and equitable (IOM, 2001).

In 2002, the American Nurses Association stated "if problems in the work environment are not addressed, nurses will not be able to sufficiently protect patients" (ANA, 2002). The impact of nursing staffing upon patient safety has been clearly demonstrated (Needleman & Buerhaus, 2003). The healthcare industry must address the adverse effects on nurses and patient safety of inadequate staffing, healthcare errors, episodes of failure to rescue, and the looming nursing shortage.

Nursing as a profession continues to address ongoing issues around entry into practice, the autonomy of advanced practice, continued competency, multistate licensure, and the appropriate educational credential for professional certification.

Registered nurses as lifelong learners must have available the appropriate and adequate professional development and continuing education opportunities to maintain and advance skills and enhance competencies. Such a positive climate promotes mentoring and speeds the transition of the registered nurse from novice to expert. Significant variation in employers' support for the professional development of nurse employees forces registered nurses to find innovative learning solutions, and may even prompt migration to another nursing environment that values and encourages the contributions of the lifelong learner.

Whatever the practice venue, in the next decade, registered nurses will continue to partner with others to seek to advance the nation's health through many initiatives, such as meeting the goals of Healthy People 2010 to increase the quality and years of healthy life and eliminate health disparities. Such partnerships truly reflect the definition of nursing and illustrate the essential features of contemporary nursing practice:

- Provision of a caring relationship that facilitates health and healing.

- Attention to the range of human experiences and responses to health, disease, and illness within the physical and social environments.

- Integration of objective data with knowledge gained from an appreciation of the patient's or group's subjective experience.

- Application of scientific knowledge to the processes of diagnosis and treatment through the use of judgment and critical thinking.

- Advancement of professional nursing knowledge through scholarly inquiry.

- Influence of social and public policy to promote social justice.
(*Nursing's Social Policy Statement*, 2003)

STANDARDS OF NURSING PRACTICE

STANDARDS OF PRACTICE

STANDARD 1. ASSESSMENT

The registered nurse collects comprehensive data pertinent to the patient's health or the situation.

Measurement Criteria:

The registered nurse:

- Collects data in a systematic and ongoing process.

- Involves the patient, family, other healthcare providers, and environment, as appropriate, in holistic data collection.

- Prioritizes data collection activities based on the patient's immediate condition, or anticipated needs of the patient or situation.

- Uses appropriate evidence-based assessment techniques and instruments in collecting pertinent data.

- Uses analytical models and problem-solving tools.

- Synthesizes available data, information, and knowledge relevant to the situation to identify patterns and variances.

- Documents relevant data in a retrievable format.

Additional Measurement Criteria for the Advanced Practice Registered Nurse:

The advanced practice registered nurse:

- Initiates and interprets diagnostic tests and procedures relevant to the patient's current status.

STANDARD 2. DIAGNOSIS

The registered nurse analyzes the assessment data to determine the diagnoses or issues.

Measurement Criteria:

The registered nurse:

- Derives the diagnoses or issues based on assessment data.

- Validates the diagnoses or issues with the patient, family, and other healthcare providers when possible and appropriate.

- Documents diagnoses or issues in a manner that facilitates the determination of the expected outcomes and plan.

Additional Measurement Criteria for the Advanced Practice Registered Nurse:

The advanced practice registered nurse:

- Systematically compares and contrasts clinical findings with normal and abnormal variations and developmental events in formulating a differential diagnosis.

- Utilizes complex data and information obtained during interview, examination, and diagnostic procedures in identifying diagnoses.

- Assists staff in developing and maintaining competency in the diagnostic process.

STANDARD 3. OUTCOMES IDENTIFICATION

The registered nurse identifies expected outcomes for a plan individualized to the patient or the situation.

Measurement Criteria:

The registered nurse:

- Involves the patient, family, and other healthcare providers in formulating expected outcomes when possible and appropriate.

- Derives culturally appropriate expected outcomes from the diagnoses.

- Considers associated risks, benefits, costs, current scientific evidence, and clinical expertise when formulating expected outcomes.

- Defines expected outcomes in terms of the patient, patient values, ethical considerations, environment, or situation with such consideration as associated risks, benefits and costs, and current scientific evidence.

- Includes a time estimate for attainment of expected outcomes.

- Develops expected outcomes that provide direction for continuity of care.

- Modifies expected outcomes based on changes in the status of the patient or evaluation of the situation.

- Documents expected outcomes as measurable goals.

Additional Measurement Criteria for the Advanced Practice Registered Nurse:

The advanced practice registered nurse:

- Identifies expected outcomes that incorporate scientific evidence and are achievable through implementation of evidence-based practices.

- Identifies expected outcomes that incorporate cost and clinical effectiveness, patient satisfaction, and continuity and consistency among providers.

- Supports the use of clinical guidelines linked to positive patient outcomes.

STANDARD 4. PLANNING

The registered nurse develops a plan that prescribes strategies and alternatives to attain expected outcomes.

Measurement Criteria:

The registered nurse:

- Develops an individualized plan considering patient characteristics or the situation (e.g., age and culturally appropriate, environmentally sensitive).

- Develops the plan in conjunction with the patient, family, and others, as appropriate.

- Includes strategies within the plan that address each of the identified diagnoses or issues, which may include strategies for promotion and restoration of health and prevention of illness, injury, and disease.

- Provides for continuity within the plan.

- Incorporates an implementation pathway or timeline within the plan.

- Establishes the plan priorities with the patient, family, and others as appropriate.

- Utilizes the plan to provide direction to other members of the healthcare team.

- Defines the plan to reflect current statutes, rules and regulations, and standards.

- Integrates current trends and research affecting care in the planning process.

- Considers the economic impact of the plan.

- Uses standardized language or recognized terminology to document the plan.

Additional Measurement Criteria for the Advanced Practice Registered Nurse:

The advanced practice registered nurse:

- Identifies assessment, diagnostic strategies, and therapeutic interventions within the plan that reflect current evidence, including data, research, literature, and expert clinical knowledge.

- Selects or designs strategies to meet the multifaceted needs of complex patients.

- Includes the synthesis of patients' values and beliefs regarding nursing and medical therapies within the plan.

Additional Measurement Criteria for the Nursing Role Specialty:

The registered nurse in a nursing role specialty:

- Participates in the design and development of multidisciplinary and interdisciplinary processes to address the situation or issue.

- Contributes to the development and continuous improvement of organizational systems that support the planning process.

- Supports the integration of clinical, human, and financial resources to enhance and complete the decision-making processes.

STANDARD 5. IMPLEMENTATION

The registered nurse implements the identified plan.

Measurement Criteria:

The registered nurse:

- Implements the plan in a safe and timely manner.
- Documents implementation and any modifications, including changes or omissions, of the identified plan.
- Utilizes evidence-based interventions and treatments specific to the diagnosis or problem.
- Utilizes community resources and systems to implement the plan.
- Collaborates with nursing colleagues and others to implement the plan.

Additional Measurement Criteria for the Advanced Practice Registered Nurse:

The advanced practice registered nurse:

- Facilitates utilization of systems and community resources to implement the plan.
- Supports collaboration with nursing colleagues and other disciplines to implement the plan.
- Incorporates new knowledge and strategies to initiate change in nursing care practices if desired outcomes are not achieved.

Additional Measurement Criteria for the Nursing Role Specialty:

The registered nurse in a nursing role specialty:

- Implements the plan using principles and concepts of project or systems management.
- Fosters organizational systems that support implementation of the plan.

STANDARD 5A: COORDINATION OF CARE

The registered nurse coordinates care delivery.

Measurement Criteria:

The registered nurse:

- Coordinates implementation of the plan.
- Documents the coordination of the care.

Measurement Criteria for the Advanced Practice Registered Nurse:

The advanced practice registered nurse:

- Provides leadership in the coordination of multidisciplinary health care for integrated delivery of patient care services.
- Synthesizes data and information to prescribe necessary system and community support measures, including environmental modifications.
- Coordinates system and community resources that enhance delivery of care across continuums.

STANDARD 5B: HEALTH TEACHING AND HEALTH PROMOTION

The registered nurse employs strategies to promote health and a safe environment.

Measurement Criteria:

The registered nurse:

- Provides health teaching that addresses such topics as healthy lifestyles, risk-reducing behaviors, developmental needs, activities of daily living, and preventive self-care.

- Uses health promotion and health teaching methods appropriate to the situation and the patient's developmental level, learning needs, readiness, ability to learn, language preference, and culture.

- Seeks opportunities for feedback and evaluation of the effectiveness of the strategies used.

Additional Measurement Criteria for the Advanced Practice Registered Nurse:

The advanced practice registered nurse:

- Synthesizes empirical evidence on risk behaviors, learning theories, behavioral change theories, motivational theories, epidemiology, and other related theories and frameworks when designing health information and patient education.

- Designs health information and patient education appropriate to the patient's developmental level, learning needs, readiness to learn, and cultural values and beliefs.

- Evaluates health information resources, such as the Internet, within the area of practice for accuracy, readability, and comprehensibility to help patients access quality health information.

STANDARD 5C: CONSULTATION

The advanced practice registered nurse and the nursing role specialist provide consultation to influence the identified plan, enhance the abilities of others, and effect change.

Measurement Criteria for the Advanced Practice Registered Nurse:

The advanced practice registered nurse:

- Synthesizes clinical data, theoretical frameworks, and evidence when providing consultation.

- Facilitates the effectiveness of a consultation by involving the patient in decision-making and negotiating role responsibilities.

- Communicates consultation recommendations that facilitate change.

Measurement Criteria for the Nursing Role Specialty:

The registered nurse in a nursing role specialty:

- Synthesizes data, information, theoretical frameworks and evidence when providing consultation.

- Facilitates the effectiveness of a consultation by involving the stakeholders in the decision-making process.

- Communicates consultation recommendations that influence the identified plan, facilitate understanding by involved stakeholders, enhance the work of others, and effect change.

STANDARD 5D: PRESCRIPTIVE AUTHORITY AND TREATMENT

The advanced practice registered nurse uses prescriptive authority, procedures, referrals, treatments, and therapies in accordance with state and federal laws and regulations.

Measurement Criteria for the Advanced Practice Registered Nurse:

The advanced practice registered nurse:

- Prescribes evidence-based treatments, therapies, and procedures, considering the patient's comprehensive healthcare needs.

- Prescribes pharmacologic agents based on a current knowledge of pharmacology and physiology.

- Prescribes specific pharmacological agents and/or treatments based on clinical indicators, the patient's status and needs, and the results of diagnostic and laboratory tests.

- Evaluates therapeutic and potential adverse effects of pharmacological and non-pharmacological treatments.

- Provides patients with information about intended effects and potential adverse effects of proposed prescriptive therapies.

- Provides information about costs, alternative treatments and procedures, as appropriate.

STANDARD 6. EVALUATION

The registered nurse evaluates progress toward attainment of outcomes.

Measurement Criteria:

The registered nurse:

- Conducts a systematic, ongoing, and criterion-based evaluation of the outcomes in relation to the structures and processes prescribed by the plan and the indicated timeline.

- Includes the patient and others involved in the care or situation in the evaluative process.

- Evaluates the effectiveness of the planned strategies in relation to patient responses and the attainment of the expected outcomes.

- Documents the results of the evaluation.

- Uses ongoing assessment data to revise the diagnoses, outcomes, the plan, and the implementation as needed.

- Disseminates the results to the patient and others involved in the care or situation, as appropriate, in accordance with state and federal laws and regulations.

Additional Measurement Criteria for the Advanced Practice Registered Nurse:

The advanced practice registered nurse:

- Evaluates the accuracy of the diagnosis and effectiveness of the interventions in relationship to the patient's attainment of expected outcomes.

- Synthesizes the results of the evaluation analyses to determine the impact of the plan on the affected patients, families, groups, communities, and institutions.

- Uses the results of the evaluation analyses to make or recommend process or structural changes, including policy, procedure or protocol documentation, as appropriate.

Continued ▶

Additional Measurement Criteria for the Nursing Role Specialty:

The registered nurse in a nursing role specialty:

- Uses the results of the evaluation analyses to make or recommend process or structural changes, including policy, procedure or protocol documentation, as appropriate.

- Synthesizes the results of the evaluation analyses to determine the impact of the plan on the affected patients, families, groups, communities, and institutions, networks, and organizations.

STANDARDS OF PROFESSIONAL PERFORMANCE

STANDARD 7. QUALITY OF PRACTICE

The registered nurse systematically enhances the quality and effectiveness of nursing practice.

Measurement Criteria:

The registered nurse:

- Demonstrates quality by documenting the application of the nursing process in a responsible, accountable, and ethical manner.

- Uses the results of quality improvement activities to initiate changes in nursing practice and in the healthcare delivery system.

- Uses creativity and innovation in nursing practice to improve care delivery.

- Incorporates new knowledge to initiate changes in nursing practice if desired outcomes are not achieved.

- Participates in quality improvement activities. Such activities may include:

  - Identifying aspects of practice important for quality monitoring.
  - Using indicators developed to monitor quality and effectiveness of nursing practice.
  - Collecting data to monitor quality and effectiveness of nursing practice.
  - Analyzing quality data to identify opportunities for improving nursing practice.
  - Formulating recommendations to improve nursing practice or outcomes.
  - Implementing activities to enhance the quality of nursing practice.
  - Developing, implementing, and evaluating policies, procedures, and/or guidelines to improve the quality of practice.
  - Participating on interdisciplinary teams to evaluate clinical care or health services.
  - Participating in efforts to minimize costs and unnecessary duplication.
  - Analyzing factors related to safety, satisfaction, effectiveness, and cost/benefit options.
  - Analyzing organizational systems for barriers.
  - Implementing processes to remove or decrease barriers within organizational systems.

Continued ▶

Additional Measurement Criteria for the Advanced Practice Registered Nurse:

The advanced practice registered nurse:

- Obtains and maintains professional certification if available in the area of expertise.

- Designs quality improvement initiatives.

- Implements initiatives to evaluate the need for change.

- Evaluates the practice environment and quality of nursing care rendered in relation to existing evidence, identifying opportunities for the generation and use of research.

Additional Measurement Criteria for the Nursing Role Specialty:

The registered nurse in a nursing role specialty:

- Obtains and maintains professional certification if available in the area of expertise.

- Designs quality improvement initiatives.

- Implements initiatives to evaluate the need for change.

- Evaluates the practice environment in relation to existing evidence, identifying opportunities for the generation and use of research.

STANDARD 8. EDUCATION

The registered nurse attains knowledge and competency that reflects current nursing practice.

Measurement Criteria:

The registered nurse:

- Participates in ongoing educational activities related to appropriate knowledge bases and professional issues.

- Demonstrates a commitment to lifelong learning through self-reflection and inquiry to identify learning needs.

- Seeks experiences that reflect current practice in order to maintain skills and competence in clinical practice or role performance.

- Acquires knowledge and skills appropriate to the specialty area, practice setting, role, or situation.

- Maintains professional records that provide evidence of competency and life long learning.

- Seeks experiences and formal and independent learning activities to maintain and develop clinical and professional skills and knowledge.

Additional Measurement Criteria for the Advanced Practice Registered Nurse:

The advanced practice registered nurse:

- Uses current healthcare research findings and other evidence to expand clinical knowledge, enhance role performance, and increase knowledge of professional issues.

Additional Measurement Criteria for the Nursing Role Specialty:

The registered nurse in a nursing role specialty:

- Uses current research findings and other evidence to expand knowledge, enhance role performance, and increase knowledge of professional issues.

STANDARD 9. PROFESSIONAL PRACTICE EVALUATION

The registered nurse evaluates one's own nursing practice in relation to professional practice standards and guidelines, relevant statutes, rules, and regulations.

Measurement Criteria:

The registered nurse's practice reflects the application of knowledge of current practice standards, guidelines, statutes, rules, and regulations.

The registered nurse:

- Provides age appropriate care in a culturally and ethnically sensitive manner.

- Engages in self-evaluation of practice on a regular basis, identifying areas of strength, as well as areas in which professional development would be beneficial.

- Obtains informal feedback regarding one's own practice from patients, peers, professional colleagues, and others.

- Participates in systematic peer review as appropriate.

- Takes action to achieve goals identified during the evaluation process.

- Provides rationales for practice beliefs, decisions, and actions as part of the informal and formal evaluation processes.

Additional Measurement Criteria for the Advanced Practice Registered Nurse:

The advanced practice registered nurse.

- Engages in a formal process, seeking feedback regarding one's own practice from patients, peers, professional colleagues, and others.

Additional Measurement Criteria for the Nursing Role Specialty:

The registered nurse in a nursing role specialty.

- Engages in a formal process seeking feedback regarding role performance from individuals, professional colleagues, representatives, and administrators of corporate entities, and others.

STANDARD 10. COLLEGIALITY

The registered nurse interacts with and contributes to the professional development of peers and colleagues.

Measurement Criteria:

The registered nurse:

- Shares knowledge and skills with peers and colleagues as evidenced by such activities as patient care conferences or presentations at formal or informal meetings.

- Provides peers with feedback regarding their practice and/or role performance.

- Interacts with peers and colleagues to enhance one's own professional nursing practice and/or role performance.

- Maintains compassionate and caring relationships with peers and colleagues.

- Contributes to an environment that is conducive to the education of healthcare professionals.

- Contributes to a supportive and healthy work environment.

Additional Measurement Criteria for the Advanced Practice Registered Nurse:

The advanced practice registered nurse:

- Models expert practice to interdisciplinary team members and healthcare consumers.

- Mentors other registered nurses and colleagues as appropriate.

- Participates with interdisciplinary teams that contribute to role development and advanced nursing practice and health care.

Additional Measurement Criteria for the Nursing Role Specialty:

The registered nurse in a nursing role specialty:

- Participates on multi-professional teams that contribute to role development and, directly or indirectly, advance nursing practice and health services.

- Mentors other registered nurses and colleagues as appropriate.

STANDARD 11. COLLABORATION

The registered nurse collaborates with patient, family, and others in the conduct of nursing practice.

Measurement Criteria:

The registered nurse:

- Communicates with patient, family, and healthcare providers regarding patient care and the nurse's role in the provision of that care.

- Collaborates in creating a documented plan, focused on outcomes and decisions related to care and delivery of services, that indicates communication with patients, families, and others.

- Partners with others to effect change and generate positive outcomes through knowledge of the patient or situation.

- Documents referrals, including provisions for continuity of care.

Additional Measurement Criteria for the Advanced Practice Registered Nurse:

The advanced practice registered nurse:

- Partners with other disciplines to enhance patient care through interdisciplinary activities, such as education, consultation, management, technological development, or research opportunities.

- Facilitates an interdisciplinary process with other members of the healthcare team.

- Documents plan of care communications, rationales for plan of care changes, and collaborative discussions to improve patient care.

Additional Measurement Criteria for Nursing Role Specialty:

The registered nurse in a nursing role specialty:

- Partners with others to enhance health care and, ultimately, patient care through interdisciplinary activities, such as education, consultation, management, technological development, or research opportunities.

- Documents plans, communications, rationales for plan changes, and collaborative discussions.

STANDARD 12. ETHICS

The registered nurse integrates ethical provisions in all areas of practice.

Measurement Criteria:

The registered nurse:

- Uses *Code of Ethics for Nurses with Interpretive Statements* (ANA, 2001) to guide practice.

- Delivers care in a manner that preserves and protects patient autonomy, dignity, and rights.

- Maintains patient confidentiality within legal and regulatory parameters.

- Serves as a patient advocate assisting patients in developing skills for self advocacy.

- Maintains a therapeutic and professional patient–nurse relationship with appropriate professional role boundaries.

- Demonstrates a commitment to practicing self-care, managing stress, and connecting with self and others.

- Contributes to resolving ethical issues of patients, colleagues, or systems as evidenced in such activities as participating on ethics committees.

- Reports illegal, incompetent, or impaired practices.

Additional Measurement Criteria for the Advanced Practice Registered Nurse:

The advanced practice registered nurse:

- Informs the patient of the risks, benefits, and outcomes of healthcare regimens.

- Participates in interdisciplinary teams that address ethical risks, benefits, and outcomes.

Additional Measurement Criteria for the Nursing Role Specialty:

The registered nurse in a nursing role specialty:

- Participates on multidisciplinary and interdisciplinary teams that address ethical risks, benefits, and outcomes.

- Informs administrators or others of the risks, benefits, and outcomes of programs and decisions that affect healthcare delivery.

STANDARD 13. RESEARCH

The registered nurse integrates research findings into practice.

Measurement Criteria:

The registered nurse:

- Utilizes the best available evidence, including research findings, to guide practice decisions.

- Actively participates in research activities at various levels appropriate to the nurse's level of education and position. Such activities may include:

  - Identifying clinical problems specific to nursing research (patient care and nursing practice).

  - Participating in data collection (surveys, pilot projects, formal studies).

  - Participating in a formal committee or program.

  - Sharing research activities and/or findings with peers and others.

  - Conducting research.

  - Critically analyzing and interpreting research for application to practice.

  - Using research findings in the development of policies, procedures, and standards of practice in patient care.

  - Incorporating research as a basis for learning.

Additional Measurement Criteria for the Advanced Practice Registered Nurse:

The advanced practice registered nurse:

- Contributes to nursing knowledge by conducting or synthesizing research that discovers, examines, and evaluates knowledge, theories, criteria, and creative approaches to improve healthcare practice.

- Formally disseminates research findings through activities, such as presentations, publications, consultation, and journal clubs.

Additional Measurement Criteria for the Nursing Role Specialty:

The registered nurse in a nursing role specialty:

- Contributes to nursing knowledge by conducting or synthesizing research that discovers, examines, and evaluates knowledge, theories, criteria, and creative approaches to improve health care.

- Formally disseminates research findings through activities, such as presentations, publications, consultation, and journal clubs.

STANDARD 14. RESOURCE UTILIZATION

The registered nurse considers factors related to safety, effectiveness, cost, and impact on practice in the planning and delivery of nursing services.

Measurement Criteria:

The registered nurse:

- Evaluates factors such as safety, effectiveness, availability, cost and benefits, efficiencies, and impact on practice when choosing practice options that would result in the same expected outcome.

- Assists the patient and family in identifying and securing appropriate and available services to address health-related needs.

- Assigns or delegates tasks based on the needs and condition of the patient, potential for harm, stability of the patient's condition, complexity of the task, and predictability of the outcome.

- Assists the patient and family in becoming informed consumers about the options, costs, risks, and benefits of treatment and care.

Additional Measurement Criteria for the Advanced Practice Registered Nurse:

The advanced practice registered nurse:

- Utilizes organizational and community resources to formulate multidisciplinary or interdisciplinary plans of care.

- Develops innovative solutions for patient care problems that address effective resource utilization and maintenance of quality.

- Develops evaluation strategies to demonstrate cost effectiveness, cost benefit, and efficiency factors associated with nursing practice.

Additional Measurement Criteria for the Nursing Role Specialty:

The registered nurse in a nursing role specialty:

- Develops innovative solutions and applies strategies to obtain appropriate resources for nursing initiatives.

- Secures organizational resources to ensure a work environment conducive to completing the identified plan and outcomes.

- Develops evaluation methods to measure safety and effectiveness for interventions and outcomes.

- Promotes activities that assist others, as appropriate, in becoming informed about costs, risks, and benefits of care, or of the plan and solution.

STANDARD 15. LEADERSHIP

The registered nurse provides leadership in the professional practice setting and the profession.

Measurement Criteria:

The registered nurse:

- Engages in teamwork as a team player and a team builder.

- Works to create and maintain healthy work environments in local, regional, national, or international communities.

- Displays the ability to define a clear vision, the associated goals, and a plan to implement and measure progress.

- Demonstrates a commitment to continuous, lifelong learning for self and others.

- Teaches others to succeed by mentoring and other strategies.

- Exhibits creativity and flexibility through times of change.

- Demonstrates energy, excitement, and a passion for quality work.

- Willingly accepts mistakes by self and others, thereby creating a culture in which risk-taking is not only safe, but expected.

- Inspires loyalty through valuing of people as the most precious asset in an organization.

- Directs the coordination of care across settings and among caregivers, including oversight of licensed and unlicensed personnel in any assigned or delegated tasks.

- Serves in key roles in the work setting by participating on committees, councils, and administrative teams.

- Promotes advancement of the profession through participation in professional organizations.

Additional Measurement Criteria for the Advanced Practice Registered Nurse:

The advanced practice registered nurse:

- Works to influence decision-making bodies to improve patient care.

- Provides direction to enhance the effectiveness of the healthcare team.

- Initiates and revises protocols or guidelines to reflect evidence-based practice, to reflect accepted changes in care management, or to address emerging problems.

- Promotes communication of information and advancement of the profession through writing, publishing, and presentations for professional or lay audiences.

- Designs innovations to effect change in practice and improve health outcomes.

Additional Measurement Criteria for the Nursing Role Specialty:

The registered nurse in a nursing role specialty:

- Works to influence decision-making bodies to improve patient care, health services, and policies.

- Promotes communication of information and advancement of the profession through writing, publishing, and presentations for professional or lay audiences.

- Designs innovations to effect change in practice and outcomes.

- Provides direction to enhance the effectiveness of the multidisciplinary or interdisciplinary team.

GLOSSARY

Assessment. A systematic, dynamic process by which the registered nurse, through interaction with the patient, family, groups, communities, populations, and healthcare providers, collects and analyzes data. Assessment may include the following dimensions: physical, psychological, socio-cultural, spiritual, cognitive, functional abilities, developmental, economic, and lifestyle.

Caregiver. A person who provides direct care for another, such as a child, dependent adult, the disabled, or the chronically ill.

Code of ethics. A list of provisions that makes explicit the primary goals, values, and obligations of the profession.

Continuity of care. An interdisciplinary process that includes patients, families, and significant others in the development of a coordinated plan of care. This process facilitates the patient's transition between settings and healthcare providers, based on changing needs and available resources.

Criteria. Relevant, measurable indicators of the standards of practice and professional performance.

Data. Discrete entities that are described objectively without interpretation.

Diagnosis. A clinical judgment about the patient's response to actual or potential health conditions or needs. The diagnosis provides the basis for determination of a plan to achieve expected outcomes. Registered nurses utilize nursing and/or medical diagnoses depending upon educational and clinical preparation and legal authority.

Disease. A biological or psychosocial disorder of structure or function in a patient, especially one that produces specific signs or symptoms or that affects a specific part of the body, mind, or spirit.

Environment. The atmosphere, milieu, or conditions in which an individual lives, works, or plays.

Evaluation. The process of determining the progress toward attainment of expected outcomes. Outcomes include the effectiveness of care, when addressing one's practice.

Expected outcomes. End results that are measurable, desirable, and observable, and translate into observable behaviors.

Evidence-based practice. A process founded on the collection, interpretation, and integration of valid, important, and applicable patient-reported, clinician-observed, and research-derived evidence. The best available evidence, moderated by patient circumstances and preferences, is applied to improve the quality of clinical judgments.

Family. Family of origin or significant others as identified by the patient.

Guidelines. Systematically developed statements that describe recommended actions based on available scientific evidence and expert opinion. Clinical guidelines describe a process of patient care management that has the potential of improving the quality of clinical and consumer decision-making.

Health. An experience that is often expressed in terms of wellness and illness, and may occur in the presence or absence of disease or injury.

Healthcare providers. Individuals with special expertise who provide healthcare services or assistance to patients. They may include nurses, physicians, psychologists, social workers, nutritionists/dietitians, and various therapists.

Holistic. Based on an understanding that patient is an interconnected unity and that physical, mental, social, and spiritual factors need to be included in any interventions. The whole is a system that is greater than the sum of its parts.

Illness. The subjective experience of discomfort.

Implementation. Activities such as teaching, monitoring, providing, counseling, delegating, and coordinating.

Information. Data that are interpreted, organized, or structured.

Interdisciplinary. Reliant on the overlapping skills and knowledge of each team member and discipline, resulting in synergistic effects where outcomes are enhanced and more comprehensive than the simple aggregation of any team member's individual efforts.

Knowledge. Information that is synthesized so that relationships are identified and formalized.

Multidisciplinary. Reliant on each team member or discipline contributing discipline-specific skills.

Patient. Recipient of nursing practice. The term *patient* is used to provide consistency and brevity, bearing in mind that other terms, such as *client, individual, resident, family, groups, communities,* or *populations,* might be better choices in some instances. When the patient is an individual, the focus is on the health state, problems, or needs of the individual. When the patient is a family or group, the focus is on the health state of the unit as a whole or the reciprocal effects of the individual's health state on the other members of the unit. When the patient is a community or population, the focus is on personal and environmental health and the health risks of the community or population.

Peer review. A collegial, systematic, and periodic process by which registered nurses are held accountable for practice and which fosters the refinement of one's knowledge, skills, and decision-making at all levels and in all areas of practice.

Plan. A comprehensive outline of the components that need to be addressed to attain expected outcomes.

Quality of care. The degree to which health services for patients, families, groups, communities, or populations increase the likelihood of desired outcomes, and are consistent with current professional knowledge.

Situation. A set of circumstances, conditions, or events.

Standard. An authoritative statement defined and promoted by the profession by which the quality of practice, service, or education can be evaluated.

Strategy. A plan of action to achieve a major overall goal.

REFERENCES

Aiken, L. H., Clarke, S. P., Sloane, D. M., Sochalski, J., & Silber, J. H. (2002). Hospital registered nurse staffing and patient mortality, nurse burnout, and job dissatisfaction. *The Journal of the American Medical Association, 288* (16), 1987–1993.

American Nurses Association. (2003). *Nursing's social policy statement.* Washington, DC: Nursesbooks.org.

American Nurses Association. (2002). *Nursing's agenda for the future: A call to the nation.* Washington, DC: American Nurses Association.

American Nurses Association. (2001). *Code of ethics for nursing with interpretive statements.* Washington, DC: American Nurses Publishing.

American Nurses Association. (1998). *Standards of clinical nursing practice, 2nd edition.* Washington, DC: American Nurses Publishing.

American Nurses Association. (1996). *Scope and standards of advanced practice registered nursing.* Washington, DC: American Nurses Publishing.

American Nurses Association. (1995). *Nursing's social policy statement.* Washington, DC: American Nurses Publishing.

American Nurses Association. (1991). *Standards of clinical nursing practice.* Washington, DC: American Nurses Publishing.

American Nurses Association. (1987). *The scope of nursing practice.* Kansas City, MO: American Nurses Publishing.

American Nurses Association. (1973). *Standards of nursing practice.* Kansas City, MO: American Nurses Association.

Benner, P. (1982). From novice to expert. *American Journal of Nursing,* 82(3), 402–407

Chaffee, M. W., & Mills, M. E. C. (2001). Navy medicine: A health care leadership blueprint for the future. *Military Medicine,* 166 (3), 240–247.

George, J. (2002) *Nursing theories: The base for professional nursing practice.* Upper Saddle River, NJ: Prentice Hall.

Grant, A. B., and Massey, V. H. (1999). *Nursing leadership, management and research.* Springhouse, PA: Springhouse Corporation.

Institute of Medicine. (2000). *To err is human: Building a safer health system.* Washington, DC: National Academy Press.

Institute of Medicine. (2001). *Crossing the quality chasm: A new health system for the 21st century.* Summary. Washington, DC: National Academy Press. 2–4.

Kennedy, R. (2003). The nursing shortage and the role of technology. *Nursing Outlook,* 51, 533–534.

Needleman, J., and Buerhaus, P. (2003). Nurse staffing and patient safety: Current knowledge and implications for action. *International Journal for Quality in Health Care,* 15(4), 275–277.

Nightingale, F. (1859; reprinted 1926). *Notes on nursing: What it is, and what it is not.* New York: D. Appleton and Company

U.S. Department of Health and Human Services. (2002). *The registered nurse population: Findings from the National Sample Survey of Registered Nurses, March 2000.* Washington, DC: Health Resources and Services Administration, Bureau of Health Professions, Division of Nursing.

Index

Note: Entries designated with [2004] indicates an entry from *Nursing: Scope and Standards of Practice*. That information is not current, and is of historical value only.

Planning in nursing practice (*continued*)
science of nursing and, 22
Standard of Practice, 36–37
[2004], 122–123

Policies in nursing practice, 5, 18
assessment and, 33
evaluation and, 46
institutional, 5, 9
leadership and, 55
and procedures, 5, 9, 46, 52
quality of practice and, 52
science of nursing and, 27
social justice and, 29

Policies and procedures
(institutional), 5, 9

Population-based health care
CNL role and, 20
as focus of care and practice, 1, 2, 4,
5, 15, 23
See also Diversity; Healthcare
consumer

Practice settings. *See* Environments for
nursing practice; Work environments

Procedures and policies, 5, 9, 46, 52
See also Test, procedures, and
protocols

Prescriptive authority and treatment
Standard of Practice, 44
[2004], 121

Preventive practice in healthcare, 23, 26,
27
competencies involving, 36, 41, 42, 54
errors, 5, 7, 28, 54
See also Risk management

Privacy. *See* Confidentiality

Procedures. *See* Tests, procedures, and
protocols

Professional competence in nursing
practice. *See* Competence and
competencies in nursing practice

Professional development and continuing
education, 13, 24, 28, 29, 30
See also Education of nurses

Professional performance. *See*
Professional practice evaluation;
Standards of Professional Performance

Professional practice evaluation
Standard of Professional Performance,
59–60
[2004], 134
See also Peer review

Professional role competence. *See*
Competence and competencies in
nursing practice

Promotive nursing practice, 1, 4, 23, 25,
26, 29, 30
evidence-based practice and, 17, 51
See also Health teaching and health
promotion

Q

Quality in health care and nursing practice
collegiality and, 21
defined, 67
healthy practice environments and, 5
IOM influences on, 21–22
nursing's social contract and, 24
work environments and, 6
See also Quality of practice

Quality improvement in nursing practice,
16, 29
in competencies, 47, 52, 53
See also Quality of practice

Quality of practice
coordination of care and, 40
ethics and, 23, 47
evidence-based practice and research
and, 16
indicators of (NDNQI's), 22
interprofessional teamwork and, 16,
24
leadership and, 57, 58
nursing process and, 4
practice environments and, 5, 7, 8
practice regulation and, 8
resource utilization and, 60

work environments and, 6
Standard of Professional
Performance, 52–53
[2004], 131–132

R

Recipient of care. *See* Healthcare
consumer

Reflexive learning and professional
competence, 12
See also Learning in professional
nursing

Registered Nurses (RNs),
competencies for, 32, 34, 36, 38, 40,
41, 45, 47, 49, 52, 54, 55, 57, 59,
60, 61
defined, 67
licensure and education, 18–19
See also Nursing;

Regulation of nursing practice
agencies and, 11
competence and, 11
Consensus Model for APRN
Regulation, 18
model of levels of, 7–8
responsibilities for, 12, 28
self-regulation, 24
See also Laws, statutes, and regulations

Research in nursing practice, 15, 16
Standard of Professional Performance
[2004], 138–139
See also Evidence-based practice and
research

Resource utilization
competence and, 13
ethical concerns, 24
implementation and, 38
information resources, 41
nursing practice context, 22
Standard of Professional Performance,
60
[2004], 141–141

Responsibility in nursing practice, 12
for competence, 12, 28
delegation as transfer of, 64
nurses', 12, 24, 28
organizational and institutional, 6,
12
shared, 12, 28
See also Accountability

Risk management in nursing practice, 35,
41–42, 48, 54, 61

Role specialties in nursing practice
[2004], 114
See also Specialty nursing practice

S

Safe staffing, 17
See also Staffing levels

Safety issues in health care
advocacy, 20
nursing practice context, 24–25, 27
work environments and, 7, 21–22
See also Quality of practice

Scientific knowledge in nursing practice.
21–22
judgment and, 29
See also Body of knowledge; Critical
thinking; Evidence-based practice
and research; Knowledge, skills,
abilities, and judgment

Scope of Nursing Practice, 1–31
core practice components, 1–9
defined, 67
development of nursing, 14–26
knowledge `of nursing, 22–25
professional competence, 3, 12–14
professional trends and issues, 26–29
professional standards, 1–2, 9–11
societal and ethical aspects, 4–5, 20,
24–26
speciality and advanced practice, 8–9,
17–19
[2004], 105–118

nursing process and, 3
Professional Practice Evaluation, 59
Quality of Practice, 52–53
Resource Utilization, 60
[2004], 131–143

Synthesis. *See* Critical thinking, analysis, and synthesis

T

Teaching. *See* Health teaching and health promotion

Teams and teamwork in nursing practice. *See* Interprofessional health care

Technology and nursing practice
data and information, 20, 38, 41
documentation, 28
trends, 18, 27, 28
work environments and, 28

Telecommunications and nursing practice, 87

Tenets of nursing practice, 3–4

Tests, procedures, and protocols
assessment and, 33
evaluation and, 46
prescriptive authority and treatment, 44

Texas Board of Nurse Examiners
on professional role competence, 82

Theories and theory in nursing
of caring, 24–25
of knowledge, 15–16
See also Models and frameworks

Timeline of nursing professional development, 87–89

Transformational leadership, 6, 7

V

Values, attitudes, and beliefs of healthcare consumers. *See* Cultural competence

W

Work environments for nursing practice, 24
collaboration and,57
education and, 45
IOM influences on, 21–22
models for healthy and safe, 5–7
quality of care and, 5
technology and, 28